WE ARE
WHAT WE EAT

WE ARE
WHAT WE EAT

A SLOW FOOD MANIFESTO

Alice Waters

with Bob Carrau and
Cristina Mueller

PENGUIN PRESS   NEW YORK   2021

PENGUIN PRESS
An imprint of Penguin Random House LLC
penguinrandomhouse.com

Photograph credits: *Pages 14, 96, 134, 148, 162:* Courtesy of Bob Carrau;
24: iStock/carlosdelacalle; *32:* Courtesy of Avocados from Mexico;
44: Courtesy of Sue Murphy; *58:* British Retail Photography/Alamy Stock Photo;
68: Via Wikimedia Commons, by Takoradee; *80:* iStock/branex;
108: Courtesy of Carla Malloy, Elder Flat Farm, Los Alamos, CA;
120: Courtesy of Megan Myers of Creek Street Farm; *172:* iStock/MoMorad

LIBRARY OF CONGRESS CONTROL NUMBER: 2021008353

ISBN 9780525561538 (hardcover)
ISBN 9780525561545 (ebook)

Printed in the United States of America
1st Printing

Designed by Amanda Dewey

For my dear friend Carlo Petrini,
founder of the Slow Food movement

CONTENTS

WE ARE
WHAT WE EAT

INTRODUCTION

I didn't fully understand the power of food when I opened Chez Panisse in 1971. I knew back then that there was definitely a connection between the counterculture I was part of and the food politics of the day, but the relationship between those two things hadn't yet coalesced in my mind. I respected the back-to-the-land movement and how it emphasized growing your own food without chemicals or pesticides; we had all read Rachel Carson's *Silent Spring* and, later, Frances Moore Lappé's book *Diet for a Small Planet*. When I was a student at UC Berkeley, the Free Speech Movement and anti-war and civil rights movements were going on around me in the streets. And I lived through César Chávez's grape strike and watched how effective it was at focusing people's attention on the rights of the farmworkers who grow our food. Those politics were all part of me—how could they not be? These were the biggest issues of our time. But that wasn't why I opened the restaurant. I opened Chez Panisse because feeding people good food felt like the only hopeful thing I could do.

Things began to change for me a few years later when, looking for taste, we ended up at the doorstep of the organic farmers, ranchers, and suppliers. Because they chose the best heritage varieties and picked them when they were absolutely ripe, the local, sustainable farmers and gardeners were always the ones who grew the best-tasting ingredients. We started putting those growers' and suppliers' names on the menus in order to give a public face to the generally invisible network of agriculture behind the restaurant. Suddenly, people began looking forward to Jim Churchill's Ojai Kishu mandarins around the New Year or Mas Masumoto's Central Valley Suncrest peaches at the end of August. They would recognize them. And ask for them. Our customers started experiencing, through their taste buds, the natural differences that geography and seasonal fluctuations made in the agricultural environment around them. We were all learning about terroir and biodiversity through the food at the restaurant. Not only that, the word got around that we were willing to pay farmers directly for their beautiful produce, without a middleman—and that we were willing to pay them the true cost of their food. This gave farmers and ranchers more financial security—and ultimately created an alternative economy for Chez Panisse.

Increasingly, this awareness about food was growing in other pockets around the country. There were more and more restaurants discovering and using local, organic ingredients. There were farmers' markets popping up in communities in every state—markets where customers could get to know the people growing their food. Directly supporting the farmers who came to those marketplaces seemed to me—and many others—like the best way to participate in and encourage this emerging farm-to-table movement.

In 1988, I was introduced to Carlo Petrini, the creator of a new grassroots political and educational organization in Italy called Slow Food International. Carlo was—still is—an amazing philosopher and extraordinary visionary, and he has a passion for global food activism built on traditional ways of life. When Carlo spoke, his metaphors illuminated the complex issues of biodiversity and sustainability by connecting them to taste and the pleasures of the table. His big ideas electrified me and validated my own reasons for starting Chez Panisse. For example, Slow Food International was creating an Ark of Taste, which collects and safeguards traditional foods from all cultures that are at risk of extinction. I became deeply involved in and committed to Carlo's movement. Through Slow Food I met food activists from all over the world: farmers from Ethiopia, cheesemakers from Ghana, seed savers from Nepal, rice growers from Japan—every one committed to preserving tradition and taste in the face of the fast food industry on the rise everywhere. These relationships expanded my understanding of the global issues facing all of us. I was fascinated—but also shocked—to realize that there were people all over the planet coming to terms with the same issues we were grappling with in the United States. I felt the possibility and potential of being part of a global food movement. That slogan from the 1970s immediately came to mind: "Think globally, act locally."

But back in Berkeley, I'd drive five miles outside the city limits and still see fast food restaurants and industrial development spreading across the landscape—usually an agricultural landscape—like a cancer. I kept thinking, *What good is what we're doing at Chez Panisse and other places if it's not making a deeper impact, if it's not penetrating the culture at large?* The restaurant couldn't be an island unto itself. I was trying to figure out how we could take the lessons we had learned and the good practices we had cultivated and share them with everyone. How could a deeper impression be made?

Watching my daughter grow up during the mid-1990s and witnessing how she and her friends were learning (and not learning) to feed themselves, it dawned on me that a real opportunity lay in the schools. If we could just get to students before they were indoctrinated by the pervasive fast food world around them, then perhaps there could be a chance for deep, long-lasting change.

That was when I convinced a Berkeley public middle

school principal to start the Edible Schoolyard Project on his campus. There were a thousand sixth, seventh, and eighth graders at Martin Luther King Jr. Middle School speaking twenty-two different languages at home. I had been a Montessori teacher before opening Chez Panisse, and from my Montessori training I knew that a hands-on academic curriculum that engaged students about cooking and gardening could be transformational. I had an inkling that a real change could take place—but I couldn't have imagined the way in which a garden classroom, a kitchen classroom, and a reimagined cafeteria could transform the public school system.

I have watched our country's transition from the victory gardens of World War II to the frozen foods of the 1950s; from the revolutionary activism of the 1960s to the fast food reign of the 1980s, 1990s, and beyond. My experiences from opening the restaurant to the establishment of the Edible Schoolyard Project have shown me over and over again how the power of food can change people's lives—for better or for worse. Food can enhance our communities, humanize our institutions, and help heal and replenish the besieged environment. Or food can destroy our health and our planet. We are all still witnessing the corruption and degradation of our lives and our environment—in this country and around the world—caused by the industrial food system.

This book is about how we got here—a manifesto about the effect that eating has on our personal lives and on our world, and what we can do to change the course. This book is not academic; it is not hammered down with footnotes and references. Everything I discuss comes from my own experiences. How we eat is how we live. This is the guiding philosophy of my life.

Fast Food
Culture

M ore than two hundred years ago, the French philosopher Jean-Anthelme Brillat-Savarin said, "The destiny of nations depends on the way they nourish themselves." I have always been struck by this phrase. I used to think it had to do primarily with cooking and feeding people. But over the years, I've wondered whether Brillat-Savarin might have been speaking about something bigger, something much more profound. Maybe he was talking about the basic connection between the way we eat and the world we live in. Maybe he saw quite clearly, on a deep level, how what you eat affects not only your own life but also society, the environment, the whole planet. I have a sense that if Brillat-Savarin were alive today, he might expand his dictum to say, "The destiny of the world depends on how we nourish ourselves."

I do think Brillat-Savarin would see that many, if not all, the serious problems we face today are, at their core, connected to food. I'm not just talking about poverty and hunger, disease and agricultural decay—the obvious ones—but everything: addiction, depression, water use, the abuse of workers, immigration, political dishonesty, the overarching threat of climate change . . . you name it. They're all, when you get right down to it, connected in some way to the food we eat and the food system that provides it.

This may sound reductive. But all the issues I'm talking about are consequences of a deeply systemic condition. I think that unless we deal with this larger, more pervasive condition, all our well-intentioned work to solve the problems of our world will ultimately fall short. In fact, our work *is* falling short. If we don't face up to this deeper situation, we'll be treating the symptoms but not the root causes of the disease itself.

What is this deep, systemic condition that underlies all our other problems?

⌒—

The author Eric Schlosser, one of my personal heroes and one of the great muckrakers of our time, has pointed out that in the United States we live in a fast food nation. Sad to say, fast food is the way most people feed themselves in this country. The statistics tell us that eighty-five million people in the United States eat from fast food restaurants on any given day—but I don't think the definition of *fast food* begins and ends with restaurants like McDonald's or Pizza Hut or Subway. I consider fast food to be any type of food that is grown with herbicides and pesticides, industrially mass-produced, and, most often, processed or ultra-processed, with additives and preservatives. It could be the food on your grocery store's shelves, or what you buy at the checkout of a convenience store, or what's delivered right to your doorstep through a convenient delivery app.

But the thing we don't really understand—and it's something I've just come to recognize over the past decade or so—is that fast food is not only about food. It's bigger than that. It's about culture.

Culture affects the way we look at the world—how we operate in it, how we see ourselves, how we express ourselves, how we interact with one another, what we believe. It influences how we choose the clothes we wear, what we buy and sell, how we do business. Culture influences the way we set up our homes, our architecture, our parks, our schools, our entertainment, our journalism, our politics . . . and on and on. Culture is the invisible moral structure underneath us, guiding us all subconsciously and shaping everything we do. Fast food culture has become the dominant culture in the United States, and it's becoming the dominant culture in the world.

This is happening because fast food culture, like all cultures, has its own set of values—what I call "fast food values." Values determine the behavior, which ultimately creates the culture. If you're eating in a fast food restaurant, or in a fast food way, not only are you malnourishing yourself, but you're also unwittingly digesting the values of this fast food culture. Those values are becoming part of you—just like the food. And once those values are a part of you, they change you. You begin to have a different outlook on things, different cravings, different moral standards and expectations. Now your desires and hungers are being programmed by this fast food culture, and you may not even realize it; it's subconscious. But nevertheless, your world starts to reflect the values you've ingested. You begin to accept these values as truths: that everything should be available to us, all the time; that more is always better; that food should look and taste the same, no matter the season, wherever we are in the world; that time is money, and speed should be cherished above all else; that our choices, food-related and otherwise, have no consequences.

This is the soil that I feel all our other problems grow out of: fast food culture and its values. We need to examine the consequences of these fast food values so we know what we can do to change them.

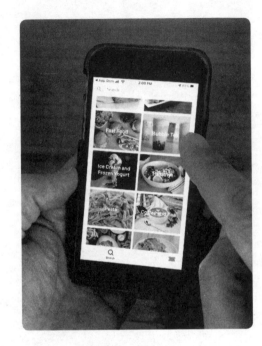

CONVENIENCE

Convenience is the fast food value that says everything should be effortless, a breeze. A few seconds spent on your smartphone and Uber delivers a burrito to your doorstep; you pull off the freeway, enter a drive-through, and have chicken nuggets in no time. It's the value of efficiency and leisure—the "easy" in "fast, cheap, and easy." Convenience does make many aspects of our lives less effortful, but the addiction to it creates problems. If a task can't get done easily, why bother? Why even do it? Convenience seduces us into losing our desire, confidence, and ability to do things for ourselves.

There's no doubt that many people's lives all over the world have been vastly improved by convenience: tractors, washing machines, dishwashers, frozen food, smartphones, Siri, and Alexa have all liberated many of us to live more friction-free lives, accomplishing more tasks with much less effort. I remember, as a little girl, poring over the Sears, Roebuck catalog when it arrived at our house, looking through page after page of pictures of children's toys, gardening tools, vacuum cleaners, clothes, hearing aids, televisions, everything you could imagine; it was as thick as an encyclopedia. The Sears, Roebuck catalog debuted in 1887, and by the 1950s it was a revolutionarily convenient way for families to buy products and have them arrive right at their doorsteps. Farmers could order their feed through it. You could even buy a prefabricated house from it. But what was originally championed and promoted as a really good idea—a liberating way to make our lives easier and less arduous—has become something else entirely. Many of us don't even think of cooking meals from scratch anymore, because we assume it's too difficult and demands too much time. Many of us don't even want to leave the house to go shopping. With convenience, we tend to look for the easy way out, the mechanical way, the "outsourced" way. We begin to forget—or don't want to learn—how to do practical, challenging things, like growing our own food. And what can I say? That process of growing a plant from seed is, by its very nature, inconvenient. You have to care for the plant, water it, watch over it, and wait for all of that hard work to come to fruition, and still there are factors that are out of your control. Farmers' markets are inconvenient, too. You might not find what you're looking for when you go, and they're open only on certain days.

When I was a college student studying in France in 1965, I fell in love with the way the French shopped, the way they cooked, the way they ate. I felt that those daily habits and rituals—which took a lot of time—led to both delicious food and a more meaningful life. It was an awakening. That slower, more earthbound way of living resonated with me: going to the market every day; finding ripe, seasonal vegetables to cook with; having that daily experience of beautiful food. This wasn't the way people shopped in America, where you made one trip a week to the supermarket and you were done. When I returned from France, I kept up French shopping practices: I would visit the little Japanese-run produce market across town, and I would drive from Berkeley to San Francisco and make my pilgrimage to the French charcuterie and the Italian delicatessen with the best olives and oil.

Even today, convenience almost never factors in when I'm making purchases—or doing anything, for that matter. I'm more interested in the personal, community-building aspects of commerce. I look forward to going to the local butcher and the farmers' market. I love the smell of the Acme bakery when I get my bread. The pleasure I get and the education I receive from those experiences confirm my decision to make time to do something that's considered a hassle. I wish I could convey to people the richness of the experience of touching and smelling and feeling food, talking to the farmer who grew it, connecting with friends I might run into. If I didn't have that, there would be so much sensual experience lost for me—not to mention the sense of community.

When we first opened Chez Panisse, all of us were enthusiastic cooks, but we all lacked formal training. We hadn't learned the professional, "convenient" ways of doing things. We were a group of people who had been educated by the traditional cookbooks of France, and we were intent on doing it the "right" way, whatever that meant. Which was never exactly the easy way. The French cookbooks available to us at the time were written by cooks like Elizabeth David, Richard Olney, Auguste Escoffier, and of course Julia Child, who described how to create a dish in great detail. When Julia Child made bread, she focused on every step of the process—and it might take a whole day to do it. That level of care and attention to detail fascinated and inspired me and the other cooks at Chez Panisse.

In those early days, we were cooking exactly as we cooked at home; that was one big reason why we had only one menu. We were taking our home practices and bringing them into a restaurant. Not only were we suspicious of machines; we didn't want the noise in the kitchen, either. When we started, we truly had no machines at all. Eventually we did purchase a restaurant-size blender, which, yes, did make our lives easier; before that, we had been using a very big Mouli, a hand-operated food mill, to purée all our soups. Not long after, someone gave us a Cuisinart, but the only thing we used it for was making breadcrumbs—and I will say that it is *very* convenient to make breadcrumbs in a food processor. Even so, so much is missed when you manipulate food by machine. When you pound pesto by hand, all your senses are stimulated. You learn from the washing of a salad, the shelling of peas, the rolling out of the pasta, the building of the fire. We still operate in these same "inconvenient" ways at the restaurant fifty years later: we still wash salad by hand and sort it and dry it in towels. We try not to cut corners.

The fast food industry certainly wants us to believe that all the laborious work of cooking is drudgery—indeed, that cooking is just that, *work*—so they can sell us their labor-saving products. And they've been very successful at convincing us. We have become more and more impatient when we choose what to cook—we want it as easy and simple as it can possibly be, if we're going to try to cook something at all. To relieve us of the "work" of cooking, enterprising companies have produced countless gadgets and packaged foods over the past sixty years to streamline the process of cooking at home. When I was growing up in New Jersey in the 1950s, we didn't have too many labor-saving "convenience" appliances, except the electric blender we used for making banana milkshakes. But there were definitely convenience foods in our house: Jell-O, Junket, frozen fish sticks. And my mother absolutely used them for convenience's sake: she had six people to cook for, and she was pretty overwhelmed with the washing, the drying, the ironing, the housecleaning. Crucially, she had never learned how to cook when she was young; she hadn't grown up in a household with people who really understood how to prepare a good meal that made everyone want to sit down at the table, so she was vulnerable to the lure of convenience. I have to hand it to my mother that, many years later, after we started Chez Panisse, she changed her eating and cooking habits and became a serious cook and an organic gardener. Of course, by that time she also didn't have a family of six to care for.

These convenient kitchen tools can be seductive. Take, for example, pod coffee makers, where you insert a single-use plastic pod into a machine and get a steaming cup of coffee seconds after pushing a button. How convenient! There are reasons why companies are able to entice us with these tools—precisely because we feel panic that there aren't enough hours in the day to do our work, be with our children, and make a home-cooked meal from scratch. We feel a constant, desperate need for more time, for greater ease in our busy lives, and these cooking devices are designed to give a little of that time back to us. In that way, these devices can feel empowering, in the same way that frozen dinners felt empowering for some women in the 1950s—and still do. But when you start making meals that rely entirely on these convenient appliances, cooking *is* drudgery—people are using nothing but shortcuts, and there's less and less actual cooking in the work they're doing.

When you're engaged with your food, tasting and adjusting and learning through your senses as you go, the experience can be rewarding. There's a pride and satisfaction you get from making something from scratch and feeding it to other people. But when you've automated and mechanized all parts of the cooking process, it's like somebody else did it for you. No wonder no one likes cooking—because no one's actually doing it! It's a cooking-avoidance feedback loop.

I think about all these meal delivery apps that bring food to your door: Seamless, DoorDash, Grubhub, Uber Eats— yet another level of convenience. Of course, sometimes it's appealing to order in food—when you're feeling unwell or don't want to leave your house because you just got home after a long or difficult workday. And sometimes meal deliveries are essential, as they have been during the COVID-19 pandemic. But when you do this all the time, you're missing out on a whole human experience, and it becomes very difficult to know where the ingredients are coming from. And besides, what are we doing with the extra time that's created when things are so convenient? What are we making room for?

c—

Convenience and speed are two fast food values that walk together hand in hand. Speed *is* very convenient for us, after all; think of how convenient that fast food drive-through seems. But there's a subtle, significant difference between speed and convenience. Why do we stand on a corner waiting for an Uber, when taking the subway would actually get us to our destination in half the time? Why, in fact, would we wait a full day to get our toothpaste delivered to our front door, when it would take a mere fifteen minutes to drive to the drugstore and return home? Sometimes our desire for convenience outstrips our overwhelming desire for speed—which says something about how vital convenience really is to us.

Once we've digested it, convenience leads to passivity and ignorance in all areas of our lives. Sometimes these days it seems that it's more convenient to let other people think for us. And yet it's a value that seems so benign on the surface. Somehow, despite everything, it still feels like the future.

I don't know that I can say it any better than Tim Wu, a law professor at Columbia, who wrote a brilliant opinion piece for *The New York Times* called "The Tyranny of Convenience": "Convenience is the most underestimated and least understood force in the world," Wu writes. "As task after task becomes easier, the growing expectation of convenience exerts a pressure on everything else to be easy or get left behind. We are spoiled by immediacy and become annoyed by tasks that remain at the old level of effort and time. When you can skip the line and buy concert tickets on your phone, waiting in line to vote in an election is irritating. . . . Today's cult of convenience fails to acknowledge that difficulty is a constitutive feature of human experience. Convenience is all destination and no journey. But climbing a mountain is different from taking the tram to the top, even if you end up at the same place. We are becoming people who care mainly or only about outcomes. We are at risk of making most of our life experiences a series of trolley rides."

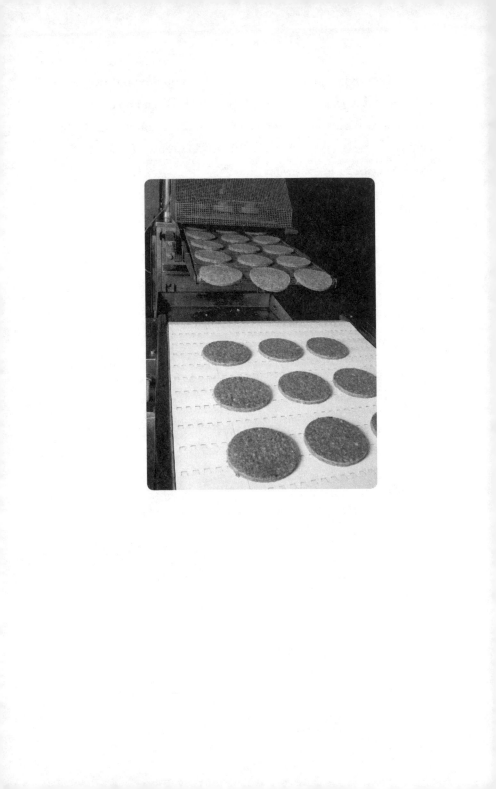

UNIFORMITY

Uniformity is the fast food value that says everything should look, be, and taste the same, wherever you go. The hamburger and French fries and soft drink you get in New York should be identical to the burger, fries, and soft drink you get everywhere else in the world. If not, there's something wrong with it, something suspect, something not quite right. Many of us take uniformity for granted. We actually like it a lot. It's modern. It comforts us in unfamiliar places. It is predictable; it is safe. But when we try to make all products, especially food, consistent and predictable—in a word, uniform—a lot is lost or compromised in the process, not to mention disregarded or wasted. When uniformity spreads to the culture at large, it masks darker issues such as the loss of individuality and the tendency toward conformity and social control.

About twenty years ago, I was asked to come to a friend's restaurant for a tomato tasting. There was a genetically modified tomato there that had been designed to be the right shape for packing for transportation, and its skin, texture, and color were aligned to a certain tomato ideal. Everybody was so excited to compare the genetically modified ones and the organic ones. There were a number of tomatoes laid out on the table, and each one did look round and red and good— and the genetically modified one fit right in. It looked like the ideal tomato, as if Pixar had made it. But when it was cut into wedges and we tasted it, the experience was very strange: it wasn't extraordinary in any way. It wasn't bad, exactly, but it didn't inspire anything. It fit all the criteria of uniformity— the symmetry, the color, the shape, the feel of it—but the genetically modified tomato was missing something vital. We had the expectation that it would be a revelation, that it had been modified to be great, but it was designed to fool us.

The industrial food system demands uniformity in order to run smoothly and efficiently. It's much quicker and cheaper— not to mention convenient!—for example, to bake standardized loaves of bread as they flow by on a conveyor belt rather than have individual loaves, with their natural ingredients and charming irregularities, watched over and tended by cooks using more traditional ovens. It's less complicated to judge whether a cheese is "finished" when they're all the same size, shape, and color.

In order to guarantee that certain vegetables "look right" in the market, industrial farms all around the world have turned to growing crops in greenhouses in highly controlled environments requiring the heavy use of herbicides and pesticides. One of the most shocking films I've seen about food was *Our Daily Bread,* made about fifteen years ago by the Austrian filmmaker Nikolaus Geyrhalter. It examined the conditions of the people working in greenhouses all over Eastern Europe, most of them immigrants. These greenhouse workers have to dress up in protective clothing to spray all this industrially grown food with pesticides in order to control the growth and uniformity of the plants. In many of these "farms," they're now using robots to tend to and harvest the crops—it's another way to force uniformity onto the food system. In these greenhouses, vegetables and fruits don't get natural blemishes and aren't affected by changes in the weather. The greenery around the tops of berries, for example, can be preserved more easily, to give the expected impression of freshness in the stores they're delivered to. The tomatoes are trained to grow in such a way that when they're harvested, the stems all look alike—as if the tomatoes have just been picked off a plant.

It's practically impossible to have this sort of uniformity in truly organic farming, because the whole point of organic farming is that you're picking foods individually when they're ripe. They're never going to be exactly the same size and shape. The strict definition of *organic foods* is that they're grown without the use of pesticides or herbicides. But my own definition of *organic* has come to include a lot of other considerations, like whether a farm uses irradiation or mechanized tilling, whether they are planting genetically modified crops, and how well the farmworkers are treated. It is a bigger picture of a farming system than most legislators have decided is strictly "organic."

Uniformity is also put into practice in the name of safety and control. The European Union, for example, has made it more difficult for small cheesemakers who use raw milk to make traditional regional cheeses, by introducing regulations that force cheesemakers into more "standardized" formats. About twenty-five years ago, shortly after these new regulations were put into place, I was on a trip to France and visited a shepherd in the Pyrenees. We spent the day watching his process of herding his forty sheep, calling them in from the mountain with a whistle, milking the animals himself, making the cheese by hand over the fire. He made one cheese a day. And the flavor of that cheese changed according to the season: what the sheep were eating, what grasses and herbs and flowers were growing on the hillsides. The flavor of the cheese was extraordinary, and utterly unique to that place and that day. Trying to force this cheesemaker into a factory-like process would strip him of his livelihood—there was no way for him to conform to those standards of uniformity. In situations like this, we don't just lose good food; we lose traditional cultures.

Uniformity reduces the diversity of food available to us: it strips away the idiosyncratic, more challenging foods to grow or make, encouraging the production of foods that can be manufactured seamlessly. The rise of monocultures is an example of uniformity at work. Agricultural historians have talked about how Iowa used to be a very rich horticultural state; up until World War II, it had some of the greatest biodiversity in the nation. And now the Hawkeye State is focused on just two crops: soybeans and corn. It's more lucrative for farmers to grow a single crop and easier to monitor for plant irregularities. But this lack of diversity takes away plant populations' natural resistance to pests and disease—it ignores the biological interdependency that plants need to be healthy. The reality is, there is no monoculture in nature. The health of the soil erodes with the use of more pesticides, making crops that aren't part of the monoculture harder to grow and more vulnerable still. In fact, with less diversity of crops, the threat of major crop failure rises, putting the world food supply at risk.

Uniformity also results in the reduction of food varieties. The author Jim Hightower, who in the 1980s was the commissioner of the Texas Department of Agriculture, has pointed out how the search for market efficiencies has reduced the varieties of vegetables on our grocery shelves. A study compared seed varieties sold by commercial U.S. seed houses in 1903 with those in the U.S. National Seed Storage Laboratory in 1983. The survey, which included sixty-six crops, found that, unbelievably, 93 percent of the 1,903 varieties had gone extinct. Ethnobotanists like Gary Nabhan have also been exploring the complex relationship between people and plants, and how this sort of dramatic decline in plant diversity affects us. Nabhan writes convincingly that the loss of crop diversity is directly linked to the loss of cultural diversity. This homogenization of the global diet has discriminated against traditional regional agricultures and healthy diets.

When uniformity becomes a part of us, it spreads to the rest of our culture, it can have a chilling effect. You see uniformity especially in airports: the exact same concessions in every terminal, no matter where you are in the country. Our shopping malls and entertainment complexes also look and feel the same wherever you are in the world. Some of these malls are failing, which feels like a good thing—but the uniformity has simply moved online. We have created our own virtual malls. Factories, warehouses, and slaughterhouses are designed and built to accommodate this industrial sense of uniformity. It's more efficient to build the same kind of building or warehouse anywhere, rather than take into consideration site-specific issues like local environments, communities, the availability of resources, and waste. It's easy to think, *The machine worked great here, so of course it will work great there.* It's a mass-production model of architecture and design. Just plug it in and put it anywhere. And you see uniformity at work when you're driving down the freeway and pass the exits with the Shell station, the Taco Bell, the Burger King, the McDonald's, and the 7-Eleven. Ten miles down the road, there it is again: that exact same arrangement of familiar stores. Ten miles later, you see it again. And again—as if you've slipped into some sort of time loop. I guess it used to surprise me, but I'm not surprised now. Every city has started to look and feel like everywhere else. Tract housing develop-ments, with their identical cookie-cutter architecture and strictly regulated landscapes, are, in my mind, the residential analogues of industrial farms.

Our appreciation and expectation of uniformity in our food and our landscape have seeped into the way we treat one another. Predictive algorithms and computer-enhanced statis-tical systems, which affect everything from prison sentencing to healthcare options to unemployment benefits, are supposed to reduce the burden on understaffed agencies and the govern-ment by removing human bias. But as a result, there are many cases where people's individual life stories are overlooked or discarded, which can lead to profiling, racial and otherwise. When we homogenize society, we forget to treat people as individuals who have different needs and traits.

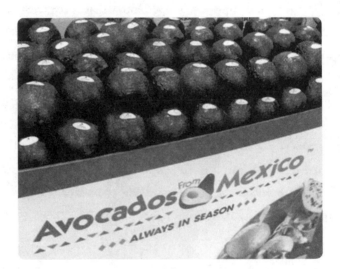

AVAILABILITY

Availability is the perception that we should
be able to get anything we want, wherever we
are, whenever we want it, 24/7. It's possible to
get peaches in Alaska in December. Evian is
sold in Nairobi. You can buy sushi in Dubai.
This twisted idea of availability not only spoils
people but causes them to lose track of where
they are in time and space. With this constant
availability, seasons stop mattering. Suddenly,
what's indigenous to certain places becomes
unclear, maybe even irrelevant. Local culture
and the specialness of what's happening here
and now become less important than the
big, homogenized, get-anything-you-want-
whenever you-want-it global reality—or
unreality. Even our personal lives disappear
in the demand for our own around-the-clock
availability.

L ast year I was visiting my friends the Chinos, who run an
amazing farm near San Diego. It was the height of summer, and their farm stand had a beautiful display of heirloom

tomatoes—dozens of varieties, varieties in every possible color. The bounty of it was breathtaking: Cherokee Purple, Green Zebra, Rambling Red Stripe, Gold Stripe. A woman pulled up in her car, recipe in hand. The first thing she said when she looked over the farm stand was "Oh. You don't have any peas?"

It was a perfect encapsulation of what constant availability does to us. Availability dulls us to what's right in front of us—what's ripe and in season and flavorful. It makes us disregard all of that. When we get used to the idea that ingredients are available all year long, we cook as though we live in a seasonless land, with no understanding of crops or growth cycles. You can find a tomato in November or January or April, wherever you are. Of course, it tastes like a poor facsimile of a ripe tomato and may have been shipped to you from eight thousand miles away and doesn't have the nutritional content of a tomato picked in summer. And is it even organically grown? Yet there it is, waiting for you on the grocery store shelf anytime you want it. When you have been eating those second-rate tomatoes all year long, you're not really interested in the real thing when it comes around. Maybe you aren't even sure you actually like tomatoes, after eating all those flavorless, watery versions. Because you're numb. When you have blueberries every morning with your cereal, you don't pay attention to whether they're delicious ripe blueberries or unripe ones. And when you take food for granted like that, when you think certain ingredients are always going to be around, you're not that curious, either. You're not appreciating where the food came from, who grew it. It's just there. The amazing mystery and work of agriculture disappear from your life.

Everybody puts sliced tomato on a hamburger, regardless of what time of year it is—because that is what we all expect. We are used to having our hamburger with lettuce, tomato, and French fries, just the way we like them. In terms of availability, potatoes and French fries are an interesting case, because you *can* store potatoes for significant periods of time, and you can have potatoes that are in season throughout the whole year. But not in the way you think. If you're truly following what's in season, you have different varieties of potatoes throughout the year that have differing water content. And you might have to change the method for preparing them based on that. The first-of-the-season russet potatoes, for example, have a higher water content and don't fry nicely into shoestring potatoes or chips. So at the restaurant, our next option is to boil peeled cubes of russet potatoes until their edges get a little shaggy, then pan-fry them until they get crisp. Fast food culture has a different solution, of course: fast food conglomerates take one type of industrially farmed Idaho potato, process them into fries, dip them in sodium acid pyrophosphate to keep them from graying, and freeze them so you can always have identical French fries, whatever the season, wherever you are, with no variation.

This is true for nearly all fruits and vegetables: while they may get riper in transit, they don't become more flavorful. There are a few exceptions—pears and avocados *can* ripen and get tastier off the tree. But for most foods, the flavor will never be anything like what it could be if the foods were picked ripe. You cannot fake ripeness. You can try to cheat it, with sugar or syrup. But you cannot make a peach ripe when it has been transported from one country to another; industrial growers must pick that peach when it's unripe and then hope it won't spoil before it gets to its destination. While it is possible to have a fresh peach that's technically ready to eat when it is out of season, it's a manufactured sense of ripeness and taste. Not to mention the fact that foods have their highest possible nutritional value when they're picked completely ripe. From the moment a fruit or vegetable is picked, it starts to lose vitality. For decades now, in order to satisfy our desire for out-of-season produce, our fruits and vegetables have had to withstand longer and longer amounts of time in transport. It's fifteen thousand miles on average from where food is grown to where it's consumed in the industrial food system. For more than half a century, we have been choosing our crops for ease of transport rather than for taste and nutrition, and forcing them to grow on land that is unsuited to them. And we've slowly been conditioned to think that this is the way it has to be.

◯—

Understanding availability seems simple. But fast food culture creates so many gray areas, it is hard to walk into a supermarket and know what's truly in season anymore. It *is* difficult to figure out what's really growing in a particular place, and it's happening all over the world. Take Rome, for example. Local artichokes aren't always available there; they just can't be. And yet there they are on every Roman menu, all year long. Where do they come from? Who's bringing them into the city? I'm always amazed by how skillfully the European markets are able to hide the origins of their food. I think it's because Europeans have had deep roots in gastronomy—they know how to display fruits and vegetables in an appealing way. Everybody caters to the tourists—who, ironically, are in pursuit of some sort of "authentic" local experience of fried Roman artichokes. But they are being deceived.

In France in 1965, I could get *only* what was locally grown. I received my edible education from the slow food culture that existed in France. My whole philosophy about food was born there. But over the course of a decade, I saw a shift happen. In 1971, the main food market in Paris, Les Halles, moved out of the heart of the city and relocated near the airport. When the market made that move, it gave prime locations to the big international vendors, who could fly in foods that might not have been in season in France; the few local, organic farmers who could still afford stalls were relegated to the back of the hall. As a consequence, the local food culture changed—suddenly you could find bananas and mangoes in the farmers' markets. Perhaps a few three-star restaurants kept their local farms, but not many.

All around the world, major cities have begun transforming into a fantasy of what the place "should" be, not what it actually is at that moment—another way in which the demand for availability changes a culture. I see this happening here in Berkeley and San Francisco—people think that California is a horn of plenty with everything growing all the time, and so people arrive expecting that bounty. They want avocados and grapes all year long—and now they can get them, even when they aren't in season.

A few years ago, Orville Schell, the director of the Asia Society's Center on U.S.-China Relations, asked me to put on a dinner in Beijing as part of the society's cultural exchange with the Chinese government. As I began planning the menu for this dinner, I made the assumption that I could get organic ducks in Beijing. After all, Peking duck is one of the most celebrated dishes of China; it's on many menus. It never occurred to me that we wouldn't be able to find them—someone, somewhere, *had* to have organic ducks. But about ten days before I arrived, we learned that every duck in Beijing was industrially raised by a French conglomerate. The only possible way we could serve organic ducks was to have them brought in live from a farm twelve hours away and slaughter them ourselves.

Needless to say, we had to find something local. We located a few organic farms nearby that raised pigs and changed the menu to roasted pork at the last minute. Even so, in order to have enough organic pork for the dinner, we had to buy pigs from four different farms in the area.

With constant availability, you become more susceptible to food trends; when you aren't paying attention to the earthbound qualities of seasonality or ripeness, you're more easily seduced by year-round kale salad and avocado toasts. The industrial agriculture industry is skilled at creating and exploiting health fads and selling them to you, and when this happens, it's almost impossible to know where avocados and kale are coming from. Avocados, in particular, seem to be everywhere—avocado toast is now on just about everyone's breakfast and lunch menu wherever you go in the world, from Copenhagen to São Paulo. Because avocados are so "good" for you, and because many children like them, it's hard to say no to them, and over time we start to think that avocados really *are* available all year round. This constant demand for ever more and more avocados affects the places where they are grown: avocado monocultures require a constant supply of water, and aquifers are being depleted in avocado-growing countries like Mexico. Transportation and carbon emissions are also an issue; those avocados are being shipped thousands of miles to get to their destinations. And how healthy are they, really—for the people eating them and for the land—when you don't know if they're organic or not?

Availability has an impact on biodiversity, too, just like uniformity. Availability discards the varieties that have smaller
windows of ripeness and the varieties that can't be shipped
easily: the mulberries that are delicious but fleeting, the Blenheim apricots that are thin-skinned and easily bruised. These
are varieties that simply cannot be available all year long, and
as a consequence, these crops are pushed out of large-scale
agricultural production and often to the brink of extinction.
Farmers change what they're growing to meet the demand.
The cookbook author Madhur Jaffrey, a mentor of mine, has
described how millet was an agricultural mainstay in India
for millennia; it was drought-resistant, could grow in very
hot, dry climates, and was incredibly nourishing. But millet
was replaced by wheat as the demand for wheat grew—in
large part to satisfy Western palates. Wheat doesn't grow as
successfully in India as millet, which led to more interventions such as pesticides and land stripping to keep the crops
alive; and, of course, wheat is not as nutritious as millet.

Availability isn't just about seasonality, either—it also
gives us the false idea that there's an unlimited supply of food
resources out there. Because we think tuna should be on
every menu, we're hauling it in from all over the world, de-
pleting fish populations. Take, for example, Hubert Sauper's
2004 Oscar-nominated documentary film *Darwin's Night-
mare*. The film follows a community of people who sur-
vived for generations on the local fishing in Tanzania's Lake
Victoria. In the 1960s, the Russians were sending arms and

munitions to Africa, which meant big Soviet cargo planes would come in and drop off supplies. The Russians figured they should start bringing something back on the return trip to make it a more profitable endeavor, so they identified a demand in Europe for more whitefish fillets. They discovered that they could increase the availability of whitefish for Europeans by importing it from Tanzania. So the Russians seeded Lake Victoria with Nile perch, which promptly ate up all the local species in the lake. In order to make fish fillets that could be flash-frozen and transported to Europe, a processing plant for the fish had to be constructed at the edge of the lake, which then polluted the water. Over time, the local people were brought to the brink of starvation, forced to live off the discarded carcasses of the Nile perch. The film follows the entire transformation and destruction of the ecosystem, economy, and culture around the lake—all of which occurred in order to satisfy Europeans' desire for constant availability. It's one of the most powerful and harrowing documentaries I've ever seen.

⌒

Instead of helping us realize that certain foods are local to certain places, fast food culture exploits this idea of availability in connection to equality. It distorts the lens so that the idea becomes "No one should be deprived! Everyone *should* be able to have this food, wherever they live!" The industry's goal is to make all foods available to all people at the lowest prices possible. In the abstract, that goal sounds virtuous. There are real hardships that need to be addressed— fresh food should be available to people who live in communities that are food deserts. But in order to make a particular type of food available to everyone all the time, food companies *must* engage in industrial production of food—and the food that's produced is neither good for you nor grown in a way that's environmentally sound, nor are the farmworkers being paid a living wage. Tortillas, for example, should be a food of equality. And they *can* be available to everyone. But the fast food method of meeting that demand has disrupted the culture in Mexico, which had the richest corn biodiversity in the world. Tortillas have long been the traditional cornerstone of the Mexican people, something basic to their identity and their nourishment. But in order to meet the world's needs, the making of tortillas has been scaled up; farmers have been forced into farming an ever diminishing number of varieties of corn, using nonorganic, industrial production models to keep up with the demand. Many of the people who work in industrial food systems live in a state of poverty. How equal is that? The same sorts of transformations are happening all over the world with other staples: bread, rice, quinoa.

Availability also means we don't even have to go to a fast food restaurant to buy fast food—we can find it on the streets, in vending machines, there at our fingertips wherever we want it. It's bottled and processed and sealed up in plastic all around us. Fifty years ago, candy was available only in specific places, like a grocery store or a candy store. Now that candy is everywhere; even if we're in a place that's completely unrelated to food, there's something packaged and sweet at the register to entice us. The lines are constantly blurring. We can find candy in every gas station, every convenience store, every drugstore, for that matter—it's utterly available. How many of us, when we get to a hotel room, go straight to the minibar to see what's there? We expect to find the same little packages of salted nuts, the same soft drinks and chocolate bars and potato chips. This constant availability feeds our addictions—we're being forever tempted to eat the fast food that's right there in front of us, because it's so easy and familiar and within reach.

What does it mean for us when this expectation of availability seeps into the rest of our lives? We want wi-fi everywhere; we want cell phone reception the whole world over; we expect FedEx to reach us overnight, anywhere we are. We look for cable television wherever we go. We expect to open an app on our phone and have a Lyft car idling nearby, no matter what city we're in. We are losing our sense of cultural identity, taking ourselves out of time and place. Anything can be anywhere—and *you* could be anywhere. Availability is creating a homogenous global culture.

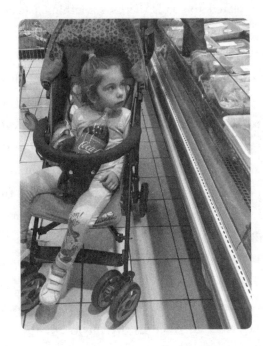

TRUST IN ADVERTISING

Advertising is the way fast food culture communicates. Using promotion, marketing, product design, branding, statistical analysis, packaging, and attention grabbing of all sorts, advertising tries to shape our moral and conceptual ideas about the world, telling us what's good for us before we've even tasted an ingredient or sampled a product. In theory, advertising can help us get honest information so we can make wise decisions, informed choices. We should be able to trust in it. But most of the time it intentionally does just the opposite, distracting us with information that is compromised or opaque. Advertising says it's okay to hide things from the public, misleading them to enhance the bottom line. It's a deception—a lie. Trust in advertising leaves you vulnerable to misinformation and dishonesty.

When I was seven years old, I memorized an advertising jingle that would play during *The Mickey Mouse Club*, my favorite TV show. The jingle was set to the tune of

"Yankee Doodle Dandy": "R-O-N-Z-O-N-I is how you spell Ronzoni, / America's best spaghetti and the finest macaroni!" I loved singing that little song along with the advertisement, and I would get excited every time I saw the Ronzoni boxes lined up on the shelves in the grocery store. It's now more than sixty-five years later, and that song is still permanently etched in my mind. That's what advertising can do. You hear the jingle, you get hungry for the spaghetti. You see Ronald McDonald, you get cravings for a McDonald's hamburger. Everywhere we go, our favorite television characters, sports heroes, CGI food products, and talking animals find us and counsel us on what to buy, what to eat, what to subscribe to, what to join.

We've never done any advertising for the restaurant. People have written about it, of course, but we've always operated by word of mouth. I want people to be moved to say, "I loved it—you should go there." And I talk about promotion and marketing at the restaurant only when I'm trying to make it better. If somebody's not eating something, I want to know why. The part of marketing that's important is being able to self-examine and ask yourself hard questions: *Are we doing this right?* It's like when we started offering a late-night menu at the restaurant to attract younger people. I'm trying to keep the restaurant more alive and full of people into the late hours of the evening, and I'm also trying to feed our whole community and make everyone feel that the restaurant can be available to them. We did an experiment that would probably qualify as marketing, offering little grass-fed steaks and fries with a glass of wine at an affordable price after nine p.m.

Advertising, though, is designed to stimulate a desire that might not even be there. When you are subjected to the constant onslaught of persuasive imagery and messaging, I believe there is eventually a shift in your subconscious—so that if something *isn't* advertised, you think it isn't good or worthwhile. When you go into a store or shop online, you don't look for the objects themselves; you look only for the familiar brands you know: Nike, Budweiser, Procter & Gamble, Samsung. And if it isn't a brand you know, you probably don't immediately trust it. Advertising guides you to evaluate the world around you in a way that eventually causes you to lose the ability to decide things for yourself. It takes away our capacity to judge something for the true quality of its ingredients or its craftsmanship. It is in this way that advertising confers value.

It starts early. Not long ago, I walked past a very small child in a stroller, holding an enormous Coke bottle to her chest, almost like a baby doll. The bottle was nearly as big as she was. Another time, I was on a plane and saw a family with a baby, and the baby's milk bottle was emblazoned with a Coca-Cola logo. These are chilling examples of the way people's familiarity with and trust in a brand start in infancy. Vast swaths of our lives are branded in this way from birth, before we're even aware that it's happening. It makes sense why people are using that branded milk bottle—because it's being given away for free. And who can say no to free? It feels wasteful *not* to use those things. But once you start using them and integrating that branding into your life, you get used to them, and then everyone in the family is subtly indoctrinated. In the 1970s and '80s, the big tobacco corporations bought up children's drink brands—Kool-Aid, Hawaiian Punch, Capri Sun—and began using their advertising experience from selling cigarettes to hook kids on sugar-filled drinks. It worked all too well. By age five, children can identify up to one hundred different brands—often before they even learn to read.

A brilliant British filmmaker, Adam Curtis, made a documentary called *The Century of the Self*, in which he explores the beginnings of consumerism and fast food culture and the rise of the advertising industry in the 1940s and '50s. Through propaganda and the use of psychological techniques, the U.S. government talked the American public into joining the war, buying war bonds, and supporting the war effort. My own parents planted a victory garden as part of that information campaign. Marketers picked up on the success of those techniques and ran with them. Methods that had originally been used to create a mission and unite us around a perceived common good were then used to create emotional narratives to sell products. Curtis details how quickly advertising spread through the fashion, cosmetics, and food industries. Advertising is always disguised as helping you to find something you want—the sweater you looked at once online, the coffee from Starbucks that's twenty miles down the road. Advertising digs for our desires and then exploits them. There is a fine line between informing people to help them and targeting people to sell to them.

The advertising industry specializes in creating an entertaining distraction from the reality in front of you. When you walk into a KFC, you don't see photos of thousands of chickens crammed into tiny cages—instead, you see a picture of Colonel Sanders in his white suit and jaunty string tie. This is purposeful obfuscation. You walk into a Burger King and you've got a jolly king right there, or a brightly colored children's play space—you're not thinking about industrial feedlots. Think about how confusing this is for kids and their parents. In the 2006 book *Chew on This*, Eric Schlosser and Charles Wilson write, "During the course of a year, the typical American child watches more than forty thousand TV commercials. About twenty thousand of those ads are for junk food: soda, candy, breakfast cereals, and fast food. . . . American kids aren't learning about food in the classroom. They're being told what to eat by the same junk-food ads repeating again and again."

Digital media has changed the way children watch programs. But these same advertising strategies have infiltrated online platforms as well, where their audiences are even more intimately connected. It's not just the advertising that punctuates a YouTube video or Instagram feed; social media content creators themselves are enticed to incorporate fast food products into their stories and their feeds. Fast food companies also go directly into elementary schools and give out branded toys for free, in hopes that each student will bring their parents to the restaurant that provided those toys. It's a three-for-one deal for the fast food companies: three customers come into their restaurant thanks to that one free toy.

This blurring of the lines also promotes the idea that children need to be utterly entertained during meals, and given flashy "children's menus" separate from what the adults are eating—simplified dishes that narrow kids' perspective on what food is and, sadly, disconnect them from the sense that the whole table is eating together. It's also addictive food, purposely designed to capture those children as lifelong customers. It's no surprise that you see those exact same fast food vendors in the elementary and middle schools and high schools: 10 percent of elementary schools and 30 percent of high schools serve branded fast food in their cafeterias every week.

Everyone is concerned about advertising to students. But the problem has become institutionalized. Big food and beverage companies make large donations to schools and universities, for an endowment or a science building or a new gymnasium—but with that money come the vending machines, the exclusive contracts, the whole nine yards. And it's very hard to get away from that. That happens over and over again, but it's particularly scary at educational and cultural institutions: schools, colleges, and museums. The institution is vulnerable because it often relies on money from these companies to fund essential services. But that money always comes with strings attached. I don't really know of any institutions that are willing to walk away and risk losing funding. But I wish there were an understanding about the cost to students' health. One in three children in the United States is going to have diabetes—and the disease is even more prevalent in Black children, who are also more than twice as likely to die of diabetes than their white peers. And yet food that isn't good for students is still relentlessly marketed to them.

In her book *Ancient Futures: Learning from Ladakh*, activist and anthropologist Helena Norberg-Hodge documented how, in the late 1970s, an isolated, self-sustaining Tibetan Buddhist mountain community was transformed when its people first encountered Western culture and "development." During this period, the preindustrial culture became inundated with the sounds and images of Western advertising. Within twenty years, Norberg-Hodge relates, many young people were leaving their community for far-off cities, in part to pursue the more glamorous and prosperous lives they'd seen projected around them on billboards and from television screens. Tragically, most ended up rootless and impoverished—a situation exacerbated by the fact that their valuable and unique traditional skills for living off the land were of no use to them in these new, sprawling urban environments. Norberg-Hodge's study is not a case against all modernization, or for the Ladakhis to remain apart from the rest of the world forever. The issue of modernization and social evolution is complex, but a fascinating and sad aspect of this story was how advertising in particular affected how the Ladakhis conceived of their own identity.

When we blindly put our trust in advertising, a dangerous consequence is that the meanings of words are co-opted in order to make a profit—what I call a terminology problem. What does *organic* mean these days? *Natural?* For that matter, what does *local* mean? Or *fair trade?* What does *fresh* mean when food is a week or two old after being shipped from thousands of miles away? The definitions of these terms have been appropriated. And they seem to fluctuate and have more to do with presentation and profit—with promotion—than with attempts to clarify and inform.

It's scary how quickly these terms get hijacked. When the food movement finds a new term that works for us—like *sustainable*—it gets absorbed immediately by fast food culture and is used everywhere, indiscriminately. And in no time, the term becomes cloudy and misleading, if not meaningless. Take the term *pesticide-free.* Or *government-approved.* Or *pasture-raised.* There are so many slippery terms.

Oddly enough, some standards reduce other standards, as when food companies lobby to get fabricated compounds such as high-fructose corn syrup defined as "natural ingredients" in their products. Behind the issue of terminology is the issue of standards. What standards are we really using, and where did they come from? They shift from one country to another. What's organic for a farmer in Chile, for example, may not be the same as what's organic for a farmer in California. And so everyone is confused, and the confusion defeats what the purpose of the standard was in the first place.

I know how well this discussion lends itself to a *Portlandia* sketch, but we do have to constantly ask ourselves all these questions about our food: Is it local? And how close by does "local" have to be? Is it truly organic? And certified by whom? For example, the California Certified Organic Farmers (CCOF) certification program has higher standards than the federal USDA Organic certification program. Are the chickens really free-range? What size pasture are they in, and what grows there? Is there supplementary feed given to the animals, and where does that feed come from? Are the farmworkers given a fair wage and considered valuable members of the operation? You need *all* of those certifications—unless you know your farmers and ranchers personally and can verify their practices.

There's an organization based in Washington, D.C., called the International Life Sciences Institute (ILSI), which has been funded over the years by the biggest names in snack and junk foods: Nestlé, McDonald's, PepsiCo, Yum! ILSI operates all over the world—mostly in developing countries—to influence national food policy by providing scientists and government officials with industry-funded research regarding nutrition. Though ILSI claims it is not a lobbying group, its industry ties have come under increasing scrutiny. Just last year, *The New York Times* reported that in China, ILSI shares the same office space as the Chinese officials in charge of writing children's health and nutrition policy. Similar corporate influence was brought to light by the chef Jamie Oliver when he exposed the shockingly unhealthy food served in British school cafeterias, alarming people around the world.

There's also the idea of carbon credits. It sounds like such a great concept in theory—you're offsetting your carbon footprint by contributing money to projects that reduce carbon emissions. But I worry that this practice exists only to make us feel less guilty about polluting. Some environmentalists I know question whether carbon credits really do help to, say, save the rain forests in Brazil. Regardless, a company can claim to be "sustainable" because of how many carbon credits it has purchased, and still that doesn't tell us anything about the company's actual business practices. At a certain point, the facts become murky—because there are no solid reference points, only the endless repetition of ideas that are hard for anyone to verify.

I just saw a film called *The Social Dilemma*, and it was shocking to me to see how every click we make on our smartphones and laptops sends information to networks that are tailoring the *next* messages we get, refining them more and more to our individual tastes and habits. This sounds great in theory, but the information is being fed to us by computer algorithms in a compartmentalized way; you get one story and I get another, depending on our tastes and opinions. In this case, these algorithms are fracturing our public forum and ultimately, I fear, threatening our democracy by disseminating information in a computer-generated, biased way.

⌒

Many people argue that self-promotion is key to growing a business—a sort of necessary evil. That without all the advertising and the marketing campaigns and the PR outreach, there's no way for a business to flourish. About four years ago, we had a big argument about trademarking the name Chez Panisse. We have a board of directors, and everyone on the board felt we should protect the name. But I didn't feel that way. I would be happy if there were a Chez Panisse across the street, and people had to make a decision for themselves about the goodness and honesty of each restaurant. It would only help both of us to become better. I want people to be able to make up their own minds, and I want them to come to the conclusion that what we are doing is right and real and delicious. If the people aren't coming, there's a reason. And you can't advertise your way out of it.

But this is the real danger when trust in advertising seeps into the culture at large: our relationship with truth itself changes. When commercial distortions and evasions of fact are accepted as natural, authenticity everywhere is much harder to discern and evaluate. News becomes "fake," facts are relative, agreed-upon foundations of objectivity and truth are elusive. Lying is taken for granted. This damages our ability to make clear personal, social, and political choices. But, more important, it impedes our way forward on monumental issues like global warming and climate change, where immediate, wise, pragmatic action is of existential importance.

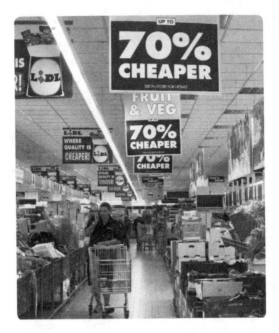

CHEAPNESS

Cheapness. In our world, we've mixed up the idea of affordability with cheapness. When cheapness is the most important thing, no one talks about quality, or how good or bad the product might be for you or the planet—just what a good deal it is. We don't understand the real cost of things anymore, because (1) no one tells us and (2) many products are priced artificially low—supported by subsidies and corporate sleight of hand. The truth, which we all need to learn, is that food should be affordable, but it can never be cheap.

The language of cheapness is inescapable, all around us: "Buy one, get one free!" "One-dollar hamburgers!" "Food 4 Less!" One of the first actions Jeff Bezos, then-president of Amazon, took when he bought Whole Foods in 2017 was to drop prices. Big multinational companies like Amazon can do that; they are able to create falsely low prices by absorbing the losses into more profitable wings of their businesses. And they do it, of course, in hopes that they'll be able to win over new customers. Then, over time, the public starts to think that those falsely low prices are the reality. And yes, customers benefit from those price cuts. But what about the people growing the food and bringing it to market? Fast food culture makes us conveniently forget about them. With cheapness, we're putting on blinders; we're just focusing on price.

When I hear someone say, "I got this cheaper here," I just feel intuitively that somebody, somewhere, is being cheated— like the farmworker who picked our food. We cannot *not* pay for something here without someone over there *not* getting what he or she deserves. We think we're economizing in our lives, but we don't realize we are causing other problems— with the environment, with our health. Which ends up costing us all much more in the end.

The cost cutting works from the ground up. The reason industrial farms use pesticides on their crops is so they can grow food more efficiently and more profitably—in a word, cheaply. What those pesticides and herbicides are is not understood by the general population, because they're almost entirely hidden from us. When food is organically grown, it's held to the USDA Organic certification standards—but for conventional produce, we don't have any idea what specific measures are being taken to grow those crops. We at least have a list of ingredients on the outside of food packaging, but there's no disclosure of the pesticides that go into the growing of a basket of conventional blueberries. And while the conventional blueberries might be less expensive than their organic counterparts, the pesticides that helped produce them can have long-term effects on the groundwater and the soil. The health risks for humans are still poorly understood by the public, too—as are the costs of solving these problems. I remember vividly when Alar was sprayed on apples in the 1980s. It took a movie star like Meryl Streep to even get us thinking about the fact that pesticides and other agricultural chemicals existed; that our children were consuming more apples than adults were; and that children were therefore exposed to far more pesticides. And what of farmworkers, who are exposed to levels of these chemicals that can be hundreds of times higher than what we're exposed to as consumers? These are issues that we're dealing with still because of the single-minded focus on the bottom line.

Another reason food can be so cheap at big chain grocery stores is that grocery stores typically offer to be reliable high-volume buyers for farmers in exchange for a lower price for their crops. Because it's difficult for farmers to secure reliable income from year to year, the farmer feels forced to make a deal at that lower price. The result is that the customer gets cheaper food, but again, the farmer and the farmworkers make less.

Fast food restaurants keep their costs low by using baseline ingredients that are generally very cheap. The menus are predictable; they always rely heavily on bread and potatoes, and of course large amounts of salt, sugar, and fat to transform those basic ingredients into something tasty and addictive. Meat is an inherently expensive ingredient, but it is made cheap by the way the animals are raised. Industrially raised cows, for example, are fed a diet of genetically modified corn instead of being allowed to graze on grass and roam in pastures. Cattle are ruminants, which means they're meant to be eating grass. That's what they do: they graze. Corn is not a natural part of their diet, and it disturbs their digestive system—corn fattens them up quickly, but it also makes them sick. About fifteen years ago, I heard Michael Pollan give a talk about these industrially farmed cows and what a grain diet does to them, and I went back to the restaurant and said, "That's it. We're not serving any beef at the restaurant unless it's grass-fed." And yes, that grass-fed meat was more expensive, and we had to learn how to cook it, because it's a tougher meat. But we've never turned back. And it was a decision that we also based on health: it turns out that, unlike the fat in corn-fed meat, the fat in grass-fed meat is actually good for you. And when it's done right, pasture-raising cattle can even help combat climate change.

Restaurants that follow a fast food formula are able to sell cheap meals not only because they're using cheap ingredients but also because they're not paying their workers a living wage—neither the cooks nor the service staff. These days in fast food restaurants with table service, waitstaff is paid as little as $2.13 an hour, and these people rely almost entirely on tips to survive. And then there are the fast food workers who don't even get the *opportunity* to make tips. Saru Jayaraman, an activist and advocate for restaurant workers, has partnered with Jane Fonda and Lily Tomlin—both waitresses themselves in prior lives—to bring this issue to national attention. I remember when I was a waitress at a cheap restaurant in the 1960s and we were paid a token wage, because it was understood that we would make up the difference in tips. This led to a host of issues, not the least of which was a kind of pressure to sell yourself at the table.

Our craving for cheapness drives out local business, too; fast food chains and big-box stores have ambushed cities and small towns all over the country. Land is cheaper on the outskirts of town, so big companies scout by satellite and start building their bargain stores in less-populated areas—and pretty soon everyone is going out to the Costco or the Target or the Home Depot on the fringe of town instead of the local hardware store or butcher in the city center. The downtowns of cities are being deserted. There is a lot of concern about food deserts in inner cities, and a big reason why they occur in the first place is that small urban businesses have been forced out by the bargain grocery stores on the outskirts.

The spread of cheap, processed foods is happening all around the world. *The New York Times* reported in 2017 that Nestlé is hiring people to go door to door in the poor neighborhoods of Brazil selling junk food. As the markets for these big food companies become saturated in wealthier countries, the companies are going to developing nations and getting people hooked. They're trying to convert people away from their traditional diets, and obesity levels are rising as a result. I love the way Carlos Monteiro, a public health professor at the University of São Paulo, puts it: "In epidemiology, we see the vector of a disease—so mosquitoes are the vector of malaria. The vector of obesity is ultra-processed foods." That link is measured, and it is real.

Fast food culture also encourages watered-down imitations of global cuisines to proliferate. Cuisines that are inherently and traditionally nutritious and economical are compromised. Places like Taco Bell are everywhere, and they are cheap. These restaurants are not only reshaping the public's idea of what various "ethnic" cuisines should taste like; to compete with these commercialized, popular-concept restaurants, the smaller and more local restaurants that serve similar food feel forced to keep things cheap, which dilutes the quality and integrity of the original cuisine.

And yet cheapness is such a tantalizing idea to our psyches that we are driven by an almost Pavlovian response to purchase things just because they're cheaper. How often do we fall prey to a compelling-sounding discount, even if the big bag of corn chips or box of cereal on sale isn't really something we needed to begin with—or good for us? When we're talked into supersizing our Sprite at the movie theater, we think we've gotten a great deal—but all we did was spend more than we would have on a regular-size drink. That idea of "buy more, save more" is such an illogical one, but we fall for it. We end up eating and drinking and purchasing more than we want—all in pursuit of a deal.

This is a delicate subject, because money is such an emotional and personal issue to take on. It's upsetting to hear that we should pay more for real food. It's upsetting to hear that the food we *can* afford isn't good for us or our families, or that the workers who grew that food or produced it are being mistreated. When I make these arguments, knowing I need to spend more money on organic food, wanting to support restaurants that are farm-to-table, I'm labeled an elitist. But this is only because the fast food industry doesn't let the consumers see the hidden costs. People separate healthcare costs from food costs, for example, but they are inextricably linked. Almost 40 percent of the global population is overweight or obese, which increases the risk for numerous health issues, including diabetes and heart disease. There are so many studies about true-cost accounting, demonstrating that when you add up all those hidden costs, including environmental degradation and healthcare, the cost of industrially produced food is considerably higher than that of organic food. People feel that the prices at farmers' markets are artificially high, but it's the discounted prices everywhere else that are artificial.

The idea that fast food is always the cheapest way to feed yourself or your family is another myth that is perpetuated by the fast food industry. A "family meal" at KFC costs

$30: twelve pieces of chicken with three large sides and six biscuits. An organic whole chicken from the butcher might cost $25, which sounds expensive—but when you use that chicken for three different meals for four people, it becomes reasonable. You can make chicken breasts with rice and salad one night; you can make chicken salad sandwiches for another meal; and you can make a tortilla soup using the bones of the chicken. When you cook your own food, you can create really affordable meals with organic ingredients. This is the way you become incredibly economical with food: when you learn how to cook, and when you use the whole ingredient. When you're in the rhythm of cooking, it's easy to use for dinner what's left over from the night before. I always say I can make three meals out of a single chicken, but the Spanish chef and food activist José Andrés says he can make six meals out of one chicken! The point is, there are ways to construct meals yourself that are extremely affordable and nourishing. And your food becomes even more affordable when you grow your own. It's like my friend Ron Finley, the guerrilla gardener from South Central Los Angeles, says: growing your own food is like printing your own money.

⌒

Valuing cheapness affects more than just how we spend our money on food. When all we care about is cheapness, we don't ask how long things will last or how well they are made—and in truth, we don't particularly care. Because when a product is cheap, it becomes disposable; we are more likely to throw out that skirt from H&M that cost only $29.99 and buy a new one. Despite our understanding of the environmental hazards of plastic, countless objects are made out of it—appliances, toys, furniture, shopping and produce bags—which cost less to manufacture than their non-plastic counterparts. When cheapness becomes the priority, it's also hard for people to tell if what they are buying has been made with integrity. Part of the issue behind cheapness is that we have no sense of craftsmanship. We don't know how many hours or materials went into producing our smartphone or our space heater, or even our chest of drawers. And once you can't imagine how things are made, you are free to have an utter fantasy that everything can and should be cheap.

At some point early on at Chez Panisse, I started to realize the real work that it takes to grow food. How can string beans truly cost two dollars a pound? How can it be only that much? I've grown string beans myself—I know how you wait and watch and water, and what's involved. It takes two months to grow them. There is the work it takes to prepare the soil, to plant and stake them, to pick them and bring them to the market. When you know and understand all the effort that's put into growing food, you become willing to pay more for it.

Throughout history, food has been thought of as precious—never to be wasted. And I think that was because we understood the true work of farming and nourishment.

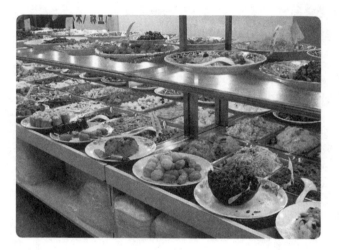

MORE IS BETTER

"More is better" validates the idea that the
more you have, and the more choices you're
offered, the better. The more you pile on your
plate, the more satisfied you'll be. The bigger
the buffet, the more you're getting for your
money. The more items available on the shelves
in the big-box discount store, the more your
life will be enriched by the array of options
you have. There's no room for discernment.
There's just weight and volume and waste.
But the problem with more-is-better is that
we're not seeing the consequences to our
environment and to our health.

When I began working to help change the food offer-
ings at Yale University about fifteen years ago, the
first menu I was shown had ten cereals on it.

"*Ten* cereals?" I asked.

"Yes, the kids like choice," I was told.

But when we looked more closely at the ingredients in
these cereals, we noticed two things. First, they were almost

all made by the same company; and second, most of them just had different configurations of the same ingredients: highly processed grains, sugar, and salt.

Here in the United States, many of us have the immense luxury of living in a land of plenty: We walk into any supermarket and there are piles of produce heaped high and aisle after aisle of food. Fast food culture leads us to believe that by having this cornucopia in front of us, we're able to make empowered choices about what we're buying and from whom. But many of the things produced by fast food culture are grown or made by the same corporations. It's really an illusion of choice.

I went on a Caribbean cruise about twenty-five years ago because of a family obligation; I was pretty resistant to the idea, but I went. The excess of food on that ship was unconscionable. Food was available all day and all night: There were grand buffets of food for breakfast, buffets after breakfast, lunch buffets, buffets of midafternoon snacks, buffets at midnight. Every time we left our room, we were confronted with massive displays of abundance—carved tropical fruit, endless cocktail stations, towers of croissants and cheese and cold cuts, and every possible dish you could think of. Everyone was thrilled by this lavishness—it was what we had all paid for. One evening we went ashore to a secluded "Paradise Beach" where we were to explore a replica of a pirate ship. I wandered off to one darkened end of the beach, and the sand was littered with trash that had washed up from the cruise ships that had docked there before us: diapers, Styrofoam containers, syringes, plastic water bottles. Another night, out at sea, I was at the back of the ship looking at the moon when I heard a big splash, then another, and another. Gigantic white plastic bags of trash were being thrown overboard off the back: bags nearly as big as cars, full of all that waste, floating off into the night.

We have an obesity epidemic around the world, and I think it's intimately connected with this idea of more-is-better. It's a physical manifestation of it. The obesity epidemic is being propelled by the fast food industry—not only through the processed, sugary, fatty foods it serves, but through the size of each menu item. The fast food restaurants run with this more-is-better idea, of course: the foot-long hot dog, the two-for-one beef patties sandwiched into a hamburger bun, the extra-large cheese-stuffed-crust pizza. Serving size is another deceit on the part of the fast food restaurants, because they're giving you the least nourishing foods to make your plate feel big—fried potatoes, starches, fillers—and of course the companies make more money off these filler foods, since they get them at such a low price.

We struggle with the effects of more-is-better at Chez Panisse. People visiting the restaurant have come to connect a certain price with a certain quantity of food. We're think-ing about the quality, but there's a constant pressure to de-liver quantity. Sometimes people look at what's on their plates and have a look of "Is this little piece of salmon and pile of vegetables really *it?*" I never restrict how much we put on a plate for budgetary reasons (you can always fill out a plate with a pile of potatoes). I simply want people to be able to see what they're eating, to taste it and experience it and slow down. People often say to me, "I really felt good after I ate dinner at the restaurant—I didn't eat too much. I ate the right amount." They're surprised that they had enough, surprised they actually feel *good* after their meal. The idea that more is better makes us think that it's not a successful dinner unless we're on the verge of feeling physically unwell. We're so accustomed to the excess that to feel good after a dinner is the exception to the rule.

I know about a chain of restaurants that operates in both the United States and England, and in England they charge the same price for portions that are half the size of what they serve in America. And I'm not surprised. I don't know what the moral is there, exactly, but I don't think it's that more is better!

More-is-better can feel adjacent to ideas of hospitality—ideas about the gracious host who wants to feed everyone, who wants to give her guests a feeling of expansiveness and generosity. Perhaps we got this from the tradition of feasting and celebrating around a holiday or birthday or wedding. But what used to happen only once or twice a year for special celebrations now happens much more frequently. We've taken the idea of Thanksgiving and projected it into everyday life. I often see this mentality when we cater events. Hosts always require a certain level of abundance on the tables in order to feel like they've projected the right message of generosity— and gotten their money's worth. And in the end, most of the food isn't eaten; so much is always wasted.

Which leads to the largest and most fundamental issue with more-is-better: with volume comes so much waste. It happens in our homes, in our supermarkets, in our restaurants. In the United States alone, about 30 to 40 percent of our entire food supply is wasted every year, according to estimates from the USDA. I find that number particularly sad when I consider how many people in our country go hungry: also according to the USDA's latest reports, more than thirty-five million people in America struggle with hunger. And one in seven children lives in a food-insecure household, according to research by the nonprofit organization Feeding America. It's ironic that in a world where more is better, so many people are still struggling to survive. People all around the world are trying to deal with this disconnect between food waste and food insecurity. Massimo Bottura, an activist and chef in Italy, has an organization called Food for Soul that creates local kitchens that use food that otherwise would be thrown away to feed underserved populations in communities around the world. In Brazil, the chef Alex Atala is trying to figure out how to rescue some of that restaurant and grocery store waste and make delicious meals from it. He has been cooking vegetable stems and leaves that would ordinarily be discarded; amazingly, he even fries banana peels! We don't know how to cook that resourcefully—we're not taught to cook in an economical way, where we understand the value of the whole ingredient: the tops of the beets, the stems of the chard, the bones of the chicken.

Our garbage cans and landfills keep getting more and more filled with wasted food, yes, but also with boxes and bubble wrap from things shipped to us from halfway around the world. There's an "out of sight, out of mind" mentality we all have; we put something into a garbage can or a recycling bin and feel we have done our duty, but it still exists in the world. There's so much waste that sometimes it becomes part of our landscape. In major cities all around the world, we've come to accept that public trash cans are often pushed past capacity, overflowing onto sidewalks. There are self-storage units popping up everywhere so people can store the stuff they don't need any longer to make room to buy more! On the East River in New York City, there's a whole block of apartment buildings that have been turned into storage units. What are we thinking? Wendell Berry, one of my favorite writers and philosophers, says, "Don't own so much clutter that you will be relieved to see your house catch on fire."

In the United States, we have been habituated to feel we deserve this sort of excess: we're a superpower, and we feel we ought to have this wealth of options. Fast food culture preys on people who have worked hard all week long, telling them that *quantity* should be their reward at the end of the day. More-is-better gives us a false feeling of having succeeded: the big screen in every room, the gigantic refrigerator, the Jet Ski taken out once a year, the clothes worn once that fill up the closet. People buy houses so big that there are rooms that they don't even go into. Filmmaker Lauren Greenfield beautifully captured this phenomenon of greed in her documentary *Queen of Versailles*, which follows the fortunes of a billionaire couple in the process of constructing a ninety-thousand-square-foot estate during the 2008 housing and financial crisis. It's an extraordinary document of how gluttony is sold to us as pleasure.

Some of the appeal of more-is-better is historical, particularly in the case of people who have lived through times of deprivation, like wars, or grown up in impoverished circumstances. More-is-better is based on a sense that there will never be enough. There's a fear of scarcity at the root of this. And fast food culture takes full advantage of this anxiety.

We don't need to live this way. I grew up right after World War II, and I remember my parents saved all the wrapping paper and ribbons from Christmas, ironing the ribbons and using them again the next year. They saved all their tin cans so the metal could be used again, and carefully tied their newspapers up in a bundle to recycle them. We only had a little garbage can eighteen inches high for a family of six, and it was picked up once a week. We learned to turn out the lights when leaving a room. My environmental awareness is rooted there, in my childhood, even though I didn't understand it at the time. I wanted new clothes—not the hand-me-downs my sister had already worn. I was pulled toward the need to buy. It was a time in the 1950s when this sort of celebration of consumption was on the rise. Ads and television commercials were everywhere. The thrifty lifestyle my parents led seemed to be disappearing. But strangely enough, I find myself saving wrapping paper and ribbons from year to year; and it encourages me that now my daughter does, too. I know that once we come to terms with this tremendous issue—this environmental disaster of waste—we can find new, contemporary ways to integrate small acts of conservation back into our lives.

More-is-better affects ideas about business size too. I always felt there was an optimal size for a restaurant after my experience of living in France: All the restaurants I went to in France were little mom-and-pop joints with room for thirty or forty diners and maybe a bar and that was it. That felt manageable to me. And I couldn't imagine having more than one restaurant; I wouldn't know who was working there, who was eating there. There are so many restaurateurs who end up on planes flying between their restaurants, trying to put the same food in every place—and very few are successful. The bigger the organization, the less personal and real it is for me. You're fed all of your information over the computer, or by reading a newsletter, or by looking at statistics. It's very different from talking to someone. To me, running a restaurant is about wanting to know people personally. I think scaling up leads to a loss of individuality and a loss of a sense of community. When you scale up, bureaucracy grows, too, ensuring that those at the top have control, and concentrating power with a CEO. You report to the person above you, who reports to the person above them. The individual loses power. It can be degrading and machine-like. Many companies today are grappling with how to humanize their large-scale businesses.

Fast food franchising, which is a form of scaling up, allows larger corporations to create the illusion that they're running individual restaurants that are small, personal, and "real." Each one can have a different, exciting, "local" feeling when it opens—but very often, the food itself is still coming from the same central depot. And when a restaurant is part of a fast food chain, it is almost always contractually bound to buy supplies from certain vendors. In order to supply enough meat to all its various franchisees, a gigantic company like McDonald's *has* to purchase its ingredients from large industrial farms. For example, the demand for French fries is so extreme that these companies have made a handful of industrial potato farmers in Idaho extremely powerful, and those large corporate farms have bought up more and more land from smaller potato farmers throughout the country, putting them out of business.

Dealing with this entrenched idea that scaling is the only

way to grow is one of my greatest frustrations. I was once on a panel on education and farming, and the inevitable question was asked: How do we scale up in order to feed all of our schoolchildren organic food? My immediate response was: We don't need to scale up. I'm always considered naive or idealistic when I say this; the idea is ingrained in us that we *have* to supersize farming and distribution in order to feed the millions of students in the public school system. In fact, I believe it's the reverse: we need to decentralize and localize and support as many different small and medium-size organic farms and ranches as we can. Some schools are already doing this, using their funds to purchase directly from a network of local, organic producers. This way, you're nurturing many smaller farms instead of the huge, homogenous industrial food system. We have a great opportunity to cultivate a new, diversified rural economy, from the ground up.

When I think about decentralizing, it's in terms of cooking for large numbers of people. If you need to feed a thousand people, one way to do it is to have ten chefs each making meals for one hundred people. But conventional wisdom says that to make a dinner for a thousand, you need one chef to manage it all. Then, in order to make each meal exactly the same, you need an assembly line. People think that if a huge event is managed by one single chef, there will be a lower chance of error. In my experience, the exact opposite is true. Teams of people working together always create something that's better and richer and more interesting than what a single chef could accomplish on their own.

Many people might argue that this sort of decentralization *has* to cost more money—that we cannot possibly do it organically and locally, that we cannot possibly break free from the industrial agriculture model. But this is probably the biggest and most omnipresent misconception promoted by the fast food culture. People think that if a program doesn't scale, it's not practical, it's not financially feasible. This false perception is a huge barrier to any further conversation and gets in the way of creative problem solving. It always comes back around to: *How does this make money?* More-is-better is fundamentally about greed.

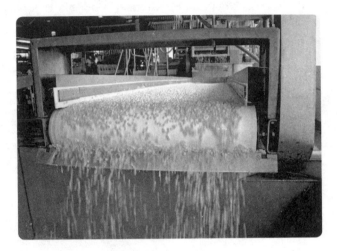

SPEED

Speed is the engine of fast food culture,
powering all other values. Speed says things
should happen really fast—the faster, the
better. You order, you get it. You want it, you
should have it. But with speed, if there's not
instant gratification, there's frustration. There's
no maturity, no time for reflection, no patience.
Our expectations become warped, and we
become easily distractible. We lose the sense
that things take time—that the *best* things take
time—like growing food or cooking or learning
a language or starting a business—or getting to
know someone, for that matter. Time is money.
And when time becomes money, so much
becomes meaningless, including our work.

How did we get here? How did our food system and
culture become so vulnerable to the pressures of
speed—and so defined by them? I believe it came out of the
industrialization of the food system in the 1950s. Frozen food
companies promoted the idea that it was a lot of work for

women to make meals for their families, and so speeding up cooking or eliminating it entirely would be a feminist liberation from housework. And in many ways it was, particularly for women who were working jobs at the same time that they were cooking meals for their families. Americans without deep gastronomic roots were particularly vulnerable, but people from all culinary traditions across the United States— an amalgamation of immigrants and indigenous peoples, with a diverse and vibrant array of food cultures—were also lured by the idea of speed. By the 1950s, many Americans weren't taking pleasure from making food, and many had lost touch with the traditions of gathering and eating together at the table. Farmers had already started to grow crops for quantity and easy transport, not thinking about flavor and nutrition. When the fast food industry came along, all of us were pulled up by the roots. We had nothing to hold on to.

This coincided with the expansion of car culture in the 1950s. Cars allowed us to get places quickly and gave us a sense of control and freedom. Eating became that way, too— suddenly you could drive right up to a restaurant and never have to get out of your car. Speed is so convenient.

Part of fast food indoctrination is the idea that taking time for food is less important than everything else. As our lives sped up, cooking and eating were the first activities to be sacrificed. I grew up in the early 1950s, when fast food culture was in its infancy, and our family always sat down together for breakfast. My three sisters and I would come downstairs and we could have cereal or toast or bacon and eggs together at the table. My mother wasn't immune to the appeal of the so-called time-saving appliances of the 1950s, but sitting down for breakfast was just what we did every morning. My father, too, before he left for work. Everyone ate together then; people made the time. But that time set aside for breakfast—and lunch and dinner, for that matter—has eroded through the decades. Studies show that, across all incomes, people take much less time to cook meals today than they did fifty years ago—and more people opt out of cooking entirely. We have been conditioned to think it takes too long to cook, even at breakfast—instead we just grab something portable and prepackaged and eat it in the car. A huge number of children in this country don't even sit down to a single meal with their family on any given day.

About twenty years ago, I was in Salina, Kansas, on my way to a board meeting at the Land Institute, an agricultural research organization. I was coming straight from the airport, and I knew I had to find something to eat before I went to the meeting. I was in a hurry and didn't know where to eat in Salina, so I thought, *I'll do an experiment and go to McDonald's.* I had avoided eating at McDonald's for decades, for political reasons, but it felt like a significant gap in my edible education—and I wanted to see how long the whole endeavor would take from start to finish. Plus, I was hungry. I entered the drive-through lane, ordered my hamburger and fries from the talking menu board, paid, got my bags, then pulled into the parking lot, next to a trash can. I ate it quickly—I was hungry, after all—then threw all the wrappers and leftovers into the garbage. And the whole thing took me a total of six minutes. I knew the hamburger and fries weren't going to be nutritious, but I had thought the food was going to be tasty. I thought it might be distinctive in some way, that the secret sauce I'd been hearing so much about would be something to take note of. I don't know what I was imagining. But in the end, it was nothing—nothing offensive, nothing great; it just fit the bill. And the French fries were crunchy and salty. Everybody likes that crispy, salty fix—and I can see why. Fast food *is* quick, there's no question about this. But I couldn't help thinking about the waste of it, the impersonality of it. How many calories had I consumed in six minutes? The whole experience was just like refueling a car at a gas station.

Maybe part of why we're so vulnerable to speed when it comes to food is because eating is one of our most basic animal needs. That drive is more than just a desire, it's a survival mechanism. Multiple times a day, we *need* to eat. There are moments for all of us when we say, "I'm hungry, and I have to eat something *now*." And the fast food industry uses that primal hunger impulse to hook us and short-circuit our thinking.

Speed in fast food culture devalues the entire work of cooking. Fast food logic argues that all of cooking, even efficient cooking, takes too long and should be entirely disposed of. Fast food culture says, "I can make this for you in five minutes or less." In order to deliver food that quickly, you need to process it in such a way that all you have to do is assemble it and serve it. It's just the same as a factory assembly line. The ingredients all have to be bought in gigantic quantities from halfway around the world and prepared in advance by machine. The life is sucked out of the food. This is the opposite of cooking.

When speed runs our lives, we become so impatient. We can't take the time to plant a seed in the ground, so we buy the plant that's already grown. We want a kind of instant fulfillment that's not happening, and that pushes us to go faster and cut corners. Speed is not about the journey; it's goal oriented. When I get in my car, for instance, I enter the address of my destination into my phone and my phone tells me it's twenty-eight minutes to get to the city by the fastest route. But what if I don't want to get on the freeway? What if I want to go down the pretty, quiet street through Berkeley that isn't so crowded? That route may take longer, but choosing the alternate path might present me with different opportunities or give me more pleasure. If all we're thinking about is the goal, it's as if we're already there in our minds, and the intervening time becomes meaningless. With speed, all other qualities drop out. The pleasure doesn't matter, the beauty doesn't matter, the taste doesn't matter, the resulting waste

doesn't matter. We think the gratification is in the end product, and so we race to the finish line as quickly as possible.
And the finish line is illusory—because as soon as we get to
the finish line, there's another race to start, another finish
line to reach.

But speed also has a little magic in it—it titillates you,
like riding a roller coaster. I ordered a special cookbook the
other day that had to be shipped from France, and it arrived—
voilà!—a day later. It really did feel like wizardry—all of a
sudden a little package materializes from Paris. You think,
How did that *happen so fast? Wow!* You're so enamored with the
process that eventually you dismiss all the elements of how
that book actually arrived at your home so quickly. You aren't
thinking about where it's coming from, or the environmental
impact of its reaching you in that amount of time. In this way,
speed corrupts our ideas of availability. That speedy pattern
becomes embedded in you, so when the next cookbook takes
a little bit longer to get to you, your first response becomes:
Why is this taking so long? You start to think that you *should*
get a package delivered from France in a single day.

There is a sense of vertigo when you're going fast and you
start slowing down. The speed with which life happens becomes its own sort of entertainment, and when it isn't there,
you feel the lack of it. In that empty space, you feel compelled
to grab your iPhone and play a game of Scrabble. It somehow
feels *relaxing* to do that. It's absurd to me that some days I

take my phone with me into the bathtub—I can't even go twenty minutes without it. I've read that when electronic images flash quickly in front of our eyes, our brains get used to them. Dopamine gets produced in such quantities that when we don't have our phones, when we don't have those images rapidly flickering for us, there's a biochemical reaction in our brains that's similar to withdrawal. We're hungry for input, because we want those dopamine receptors to keep getting those quick hits. Fast food companies know this and exploit it—their ads are edited to flash through images quickly, so our brains get that rush of excitement.

I think that, in this way, speed feeds our sense of loneliness. We send a text and expect an instantaneous response. All these feelings come up if someone doesn't get back to us right away: *They waited a day. Do they not like me? Is it a problem? Is it about me? Did I write something inappropriate?* It puts us in a self-doubting place. When we're not moving fast, getting that immediate response, we feel an emptiness. Lying on a couch and daydreaming is considered wasteful—transgressive, almost.

◦—

Our children are unwittingly caught up in our obsession with speed, but children need *time*. You can't shoot out an order to them and expect them to respond. They need you to be present. It is a gift that they give you. They want you to be *right there* with them. It's one of the reasons that Mister Rogers was so popular with kids: he demonstrated that slowing down and paying attention to children is the most important thing we can do. And when we do, it changes everything. It's funny how much we resist slowing down in that way, because it can be so satisfying when we do. But our compulsion for speed is being passed down unconsciously to our children.

What else happens in our lives when speed gets out of control? Doctors now make an effort to see as many patients per hour as possible. Medicine used to be about talking to patients and getting to know them, but now it's just in and out. (In-N-Out is my favorite fast food restaurant name of all—it tells it like it is!) There are many shocking reports of slaughterhouses where workers must slaughter animals so quickly that it creates a risk of workers getting injured. And although fast food restaurants don't want to reveal where their meat comes from, we know they're getting meat from these same industrial slaughterhouses. I was once onstage with Eric Schlosser and he was talking about how slaughterhouse sanitation workers, almost all of them poor immigrants, must clean the slaughterhouses in the dead of night. It's one of the lowest-paid, most dangerous, and most disgusting jobs in meatpacking. The production line is "the chain," and management's guiding rule is "the chain never stops."

Production often continues, even when a worker gets injured. And there's tremendous pressure to not take bathroom breaks. This corruption of speed was vividly revealed during the coronavirus pandemic. These same slaughterhouses were mandated to remain fully open during the quarantine, even though many of the workers were ill; many of those slaughterhouses became epicenters for coronavirus outbreaks. When enough workers became sick, entire slaughterhouses couldn't continue operating. Rather than creating alternative ways to feed people at a time when people were desperately in need of food, the industrial ranchers raising pigs for those shuttered meatpacking plants simply euthanized their animals and threw them away.

One of the biggest problems in this country is dehumanizing work in dehumanizing environments. I think it's born of this constant pressure for speed, which creates the circumstances that force people to work in situations where there's no room for advancement or self-improvement. Work becomes meaningless when workers are forcibly separated from the chance to become skilled at what they do. Taking people's opportunities away from them—keeping them at a low salary, not allowing them to advance or to take pride in what they do—is a way to imprison them, making work drudgery.

"Work is drudgery"—too many of us might think this way. I assure you that these days, work doesn't have to be drudgery unless you're in a system created by, supported by, or aligned with industrial fast food culture. Work, though at times difficult, should provide a sense of value and accomplishment, a sense of purpose and satisfaction, a certain kind of pleasure. Fast food culture, by its very nature—for its very survival—strips work of these possibilities. It makes us all believe that work, in pursuit of speed, should be something degrading, meaningless, and hollow. A job is just something to get through quickly to make money. Fast food culture bleeds us of our humanity; as we work within it, sadly, we inadvertently strengthen it and trap ourselves inside it.

What's even worse is that, after convincing us that work is drudgery, fast food culture then provides us with so-called pleasures to fill the emptiness we feel from this dissatisfied work life. "Pleasures" like fast food, for one. And video games, TV, hours spent online, alcohol, drugs . . . Fast food culture separates "work" and "pleasure" for us and then profits from that separation.

The most dangerous part of speed is that we're moving so fast, we don't even see what's happening. Because speed is the engine of our fast food culture, we are propelled past all the other issues in our world we should be examining. We don't have time to think about where our food comes from. We don't have time to think about why food is so inexpensive. We don't have time to think about the hidden agendas of advertisers. We don't have time to see how all the values of fast food culture merge together like a wildfire, threatening and corrupting our lives. But when we force ourselves to slow down, the world comes into focus. Our awareness shifts. And we begin to understand that we have the power to change it.

Slow Food
Culture

B ecoming aware of just how deeply fast food culture reaches into our daily lives is daunting. But it can also be a resounding call to action. Because, fortunately, there's an alternative, a counterforce that already exists. I call this counterforce *slow food culture*.

Slow food culture is not new. It's a culture that has guided people since the beginning of humanity, with customs and practices grounded in nature. Many of us struggle with the language of slow food culture. The words that define its values—community, generosity, collaboration—have been so overused and marketed to us over the years that people don't take them seriously anymore. But these values do have universal strength. Why else would they have guided cultures all over the world for hundreds of generations? And why do they speak to us now? Perhaps the best news is that slow food values are easy to access. We are all part of nature's cycles and rhythms, so slow food values are already inside every one of us. If we cook and eat and serve food that is ethically grown, not only are we nourishing ourselves but we are digesting the values of slow food culture, values that guide us to create ecological lives.

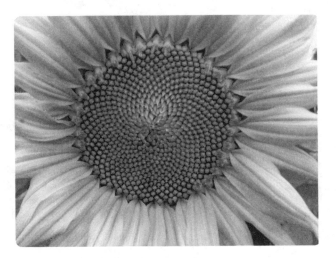

BEAUTY

Beauty is expressed in myriad ways
in our lives: through art, poetry, music,
architecture, and dance. While specific ideas
of beauty are subjective—what's beautiful to
me might not be beautiful to you—there are
universal ideals of beauty that arise from
nature. Everybody feels the rapture of a
sunset, or the wonder of being at the base
of a mountain or a waterfall. When you're
in the presence of this kind of universal
beauty, you become aware of being held by
something bigger, something connected to the
mystery of life. Beauty is in our biological
makeup. It naturally deepens your awareness
and inspires a sense of awe and joy. Finding
the beauty in food can change your life.

It is easy to dismiss beauty. But to me, it is the most impor-
tant slow food value—the one that embraces all the others.
It saddens me that it's not recognized for the power it has.
But what can one say about beauty that hasn't already been

said? "Beauty is truth, truth beauty." "Beauty is in the eye of the beholder." "A thing of beauty is a joy forever." We hear these truisms all the time, precisely because beauty is so central to our existence, whether we want to admit it or not. There is a power in it. I think beauty is an essential life force that everyone has the possibility of discovering. We are hungry for it—I think starving for it.

I had some awareness of the beauty of nature as a child. I loved the sunsets, the trees changing color in the fall, the smooth stones I would gather in the creek, the scent of the lilacs in spring. But I didn't think of it as important in my everyday life. Maybe I took it for granted, as children often do. That changed when I went to France as a college student. I had a cultural and aesthetic awakening there, as happens to many students when they study abroad: visiting the Sainte-Chapelle, reading poems by Verlaine, listening to David Oistrakh play Beethoven's Violin Concerto at the Palais Garnier opera house. But when I think back on it, that whole time for me really comes down to the taste of a wild strawberry, a *fraise des bois*, on my plate. I had never encountered anything like that before. When most people think of beauty, they think of what can be seen or heard. But I believe smell, touch, and taste are more intimate. Those tiny fragrant, vibrant *fraises des bois* were inside of me, being digested, quite literally becoming part of me. They opened me up to an entirely new realm of taste. I embarked on a quest to rediscover that sort of intensity of flavor everywhere—which expanded my experience of beauty in the rest of the world.

When I returned to Berkeley in 1966, our growing fast food culture was such a contrasting experience for me. It was true culture shock. I had had a year of living in the slow food culture of Paris, with its rich traditions of food and architecture and art. And here I was, back again. The way we purchased and ate food in the United States was so unbeautiful—there weren't little cafés and restaurants with great food and atmosphere; there weren't street markets of just-picked ripe fruits and vegetables; and there was absolutely no sense of the people growing the food. Yes, organic food was available in our local Berkeley cooperative, but it was never presented enticingly. I supported what organic farms stood for, but in the health food stores of the 1960s, the produce felt overgrown and ill considered. I didn't feel that beautiful, delicious food was something that could be experienced only by the wealthy. I still don't! In France, most people had access to ripe fruits and vegetables when they were in season, because that was simply the way the food was grown there at that time, and that was the way that almost everyone shopped. The beauty of food was integrated into daily life. That awareness of beauty was awakened in me in France, and shutting it off felt impossible. I started cooking because I wanted to stay connected to that world and its values.

When I met my friend Martine Labro, a French artist and painter living in Berkeley, she broadened my aesthetic education. She loved choosing simple elements for her home, vintage things that had been used before and cast aside. Her aesthetic never had to do with money—Martine certainly didn't have much. Everything she used she found at the flea market. And if she couldn't find what she wanted at the flea market, she would simply find a way to make it herself. She considered everything she chose: What kind of chair are you sitting on? What type of glass are you using? What kind of flowers are blooming that you can pick and bring inside for the table? And, maybe most important, what are the ingredients you're using to cook? Food and aesthetics were all of a piece for her: she was an amazing cook, and everything she made was so refined and creative. She understood that there was a beauty to economy in the kitchen. Martine was the one who first showed me it was possible to make a meal for ten out of a single chicken; she could make a small portion seem generous by accompanying it with delicious herbs and vegetables from her garden, on one of her beautiful old china plates.

When we started Chez Panisse, we didn't have a lot of money, and we took Martine's lessons of beauty and frugality to heart. The reason we had a fixed-price menu was that we wanted to know exactly how much food we would need, so we wouldn't waste anything. We also didn't have any money to decorate the dining room, so we proceeded the way

Martine would: we put it together with mismatched silverware from the flea market, high-backed secondhand chairs
from the salvage store, and a vintage rug running down the
staircase so you felt like you were in someone's home. It
didn't cost much to find beautiful things if we let go of the
idea that everything had to be new and uniform. Putting the
dining room together beautifully also appealed to my Montessori training about preparing the classroom—carefully
considering the way the tables were set and the way the light
came into the room, so that people entering would be instantly drawn in. I wanted Chez Panisse to feel welcoming
and warm, like one of those neighborhood French restaurants I had fallen in love with in Paris. I do think people responded to the care we took with the idiosyncratic beauty of
the place as much as they responded to the taste of the food
they ate.

Beauty is tied to simplicity, another slow food value, and
many of our decisions back then about the plate concerned
portion size; we were all Francophiles, and understood that
food could be served in courses, and small ones at that. Food
could be better seen and appreciated when less was on the
plate. My food aesthetic had been defined by the dishes I had
been served in France and what I had seen in the artful photographs on the covers of Elizabeth David's cookbooks: red wine
in a carafe, a classic tureen of soup, a freshly baked baguette, a
plate of ripe figs with a wedge of fresh goat cheese. I wanted
the table settings at Chez Panisse to have the simplicity and

intimacy of those photographs. I wasn't looking for food that was perfect; I was looking for food that was genuine. I have always connected that sense of authenticity to the cultivation and growth of the food, and I cannot separate that out. Food cannot be divorced from nature. If I learn that food has come from an industrial farm, it's no longer beautiful to me, no matter how it's shined up or how cleverly it's presented.

Aesthetics are not just expressed in superficial flourishes. They are guiding forces that allow individuals to express themselves. Different cooks and guest chefs have come through the kitchen of Chez Panisse, and each has brought their own aesthetics. Whether their food is Italian or Parsi or Mexican or Japanese or Brazilian, it is grounded in the foundational values of stewardship, nourishment, and community. Besides bringing a much-needed diversity to the kitchen, these chefs have creatively interpreted these values in their own unique ways. How do we ensure that what we serve is irresistible and true to the ingredients? When everything is working well in the restaurant—when the food is just right, when the people at the tables are happy, when the golden light of the setting sun is coming in through the porch—I can't describe it in any other way than to say that it is so beautiful. That harmony is evident to everybody, customers and staff alike. It is a ballet.

At the Edible Schoolyard Project, we often say, "Beauty is the language of care." What do we mean by that? When we first set up the kitchen classroom at the Edible Schoolyard, in a rather unassuming, run-down portable building next to the new garden, we began with a certain orderliness: we put all the mortars and pestles in one place, all the different-colored strainers together, all the glasses together, so you could clearly see what was in the room. We kept things organized and simple, because we wanted children to be able to find things easily and put them back in their places. We painted the walls a soft, warm yellow and cleaned the windows. We had sturdy tables made and added polished gray-green concrete tabletops crafted by a local artisan. We hung vintage posters of plants on the walls. And Esther Cook, the artist and teacher who has steered the Edible Schoolyard from the very beginning, had the inspired idea to create an altar for fruits, vegetables, and flowers that had been harvested that day from the garden. I think the first thing that strikes people who walk into that kitchen space is its beauty. They feel welcomed by a spirit of abundance and generosity. The kids want to do their homework in the kitchen classroom after school, because the space feels good to them. "Beauty is the language of care" means that when we put a bowl of citrus or a bouquet of wildflowers on the altar, we are trying to communicate non-verbally to the students that someone thought about them, that they are cared about, that they matter, and that they are in a safe, nurturing environment. What could be more important than that? A gesture of beauty doesn't need to be elaborate—I never think of beauty as fancy. It can be a hand-ful of raspberries just picked off the bush or a few sprigs of flowering rosemary tucked inside a lunchbox or a couple of candles lit on a dinner table.

Aesthetics feel so vital to me that I am sometimes intoler-ant. I am always vigilant about the ways that fast food culture creeps in and how destructive it can be, and beauty is often the litmus test for determining what's authentic and free from fast food influences. As we try to navigate and balance the concerns of our daily lives, beauty is pushed lower and lower on the list of priorities. In a hierarchy of needs, beauty is considered one of the least important. Fast food culture overlooks and misappropriates beauty, which then allows fast food values like convenience and uniformity and speed to encroach on our lives. We have become so desensitized to the importance of beauty that we forget how vital it is to our happiness and our survival.

We know how beauty affects our happiness, but we haven't examined how beauty helps us to survive. "The ultimate test is whether we live in beautiful places," Wendell Berry writes. "Wherever ugliness has crept in, we have the first symptoms of exploitation and exhaustion." I understand his point: beauty is not only a way to awaken us to aesthetics and our own senses; it is a way to decide whether networks are functioning correctly, whether they are alive and healthy and fertile. Beauty in nature is one of the outer manifestations that stewardship is happening—that the land is being cared for and protected. Beauty is the language of care, yes, but it's more than that, too. It is the outcome of care.

When we see something utterly beautiful, we enter a state of awe. Beauty can startle you; it breaks down the illusory barriers between us and nature. Beauty is out of the realm of human control or understanding, and it has a transcendent universality that can't be ignored. In his book *How to Change Your Mind*, Michael Pollan talks about how awe is a fundamental human emotion that may have evolved in us to encourage altruistic behavior, to make us feel part of something bigger than ourselves: "This larger entity could be the social collective, nature as a whole, or a spirit world, but it is something sufficiently overpowering to dwarf us and our narrow self-interest. . . . An experience of awe appears to be an excellent antidote for egotism." This is why beauty is so important: it creates an involuntary reaction of joy that humbles us and dissolves our defenses, which opens us up to collaboration and empathy.

We need to put beauty first. I believe it is important and possible to create beauty in the things we use and nourish ourselves with every day. It is essential. Food is the easiest way for all of us to engage with beauty in our everyday lives. Any meal has the potential to crack us open to pleasure and connection and joy. I know it can, because I have watched it happen in the restaurant over the past fifty years, and with thousands of schoolchildren, in schools all over the world, for the past twenty-five years. Cooking and eating food together can be an everyday experience of beauty that reaches all of our senses.

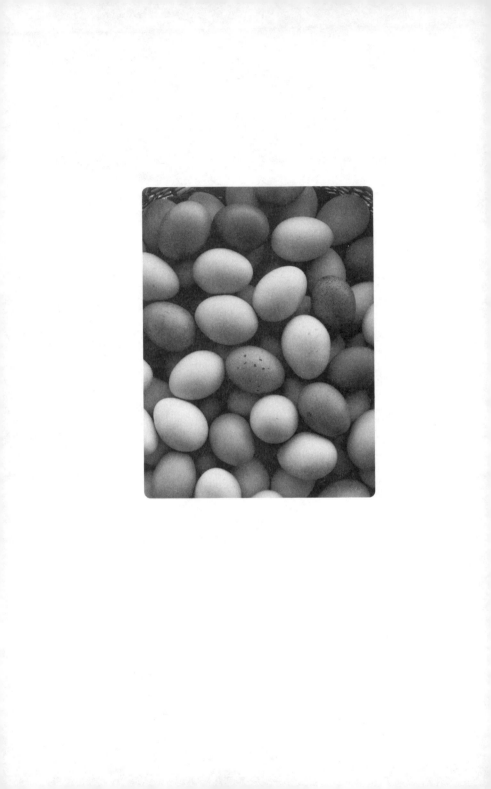

BIODIVERSITY

Biodiversity encourages us to embrace the
variety of elements in any system, showing us
that many times it's the mix of distinct qualities that makes that system richer, stronger,
more intelligent, more resilient. In contrast to
uniformity, biodiversity demonstrates how the
unique and individual traits of each species
together make a powerful network. Biodiversity
helps us see that every species has its place and
role to play. In biodiversity there is an implicit
appreciation of the other, which naturally
promotes acceptance, cooperation, and
integration.

L ike so many others, I watched the BBC's epic documentary series *Planet Earth*. And what can I say? The biodiversity of this planet is breathtaking: the many different kinds
of butterflies in the Amazon, all the innumerable varieties of
conifers, the thousands of species of bees. Biodiversity is the
fabric of the vast, dazzling complexity of life.

For me, biodiversity is what keeps me fascinated with

food. It is endlessly varied. In Tennessee recently, I was introduced to two multicolored shell bean varieties I'd never seen before, and I couldn't wait to bring them back to the restaurant's farmer to see how they would grow in California. Just when I think I know all the different kinds of beans, two more appear! Those sorts of discoveries open me up, instantly make me curious—and make me want to taste them. The same kinds of small revelations can happen with almost any fruit or vegetable: We've become accustomed to the ubiquitous orange carrot, but carrots exist in every possible color, from pale white to garnet red to lemon yellow. When you see one that doesn't fit that orange-carrot stereotype, it wakes you up. On the plate, that sort of biodiversity takes food into the realm of art; it's exciting to put the white and the purple carrots together and entice someone with a salad that, for a brief moment, is magical. In that moment, you reach them.

There have been times in the history of Chez Panisse when I've forgotten how critical biodiversity is. At a certain point, I was so focused on organic feed for animals that I forgot about the importance of breed. I was always after the organic free-range chickens, concerned with how they were being raised, how they were treated, what they were fed. When the movie *Eating Animals* came out, I learned about farmer Frank Reese and his heritage breed turkeys. My friend Patrick Martins, who runs Heritage Foods, said, "I want you to taste Frank's birds." He sent them to me frozen, and I was dubious about how good a frozen turkey could possibly be.

But we cooked one, and I could not believe how different that particular turkey breed tasted. We've accepted a pretty low level of taste when it comes to our animals: they've been bred to be uniformly big, fat, and low-maintenance, all to fit the industrial agricultural convenience model. While we absolutely need to focus on how humanely animals are raised and how they are fed, we also need to appreciate and preserve heritage breeds. At the Edible Schoolyard, we have six or seven different breeds of chickens wandering around the garden, laying beautiful eggs of different colors: blue ones, pale brown ones, spotted ones. When the children find them, they're fascinated by the range of egg colors they've never seen before. They appeal to children more and, of course, they taste much better than conventional eggs.

⌒—

Terroir is a French term traditionally used to describe how certain grapes excel in certain soils and climates, affecting the taste of the wine made from them. Terroir is about the marriage of an individual plant variety and the particular earth it's grown in. Each place expresses a very singular quality: the pinot noir grape that might have a certain taste when it's grown in central Oregon has a noticeably different expression when it's grown in the volcanic soil of Sicily. People often ask me questions like "What's your favorite tomato?" My answer is a dry-farmed Early Girl grown at Green and

Red Vineyard, on the east side of California's Pope Valley, in the heat of August. I know this sounds overly specific. But it's true: that tomato variety has a unique expression there, in that place, at that time. Dry-farmed Early Girl tomatoes from Dirty Girl Produce are very special, too—grown down in Half Moon Bay, right near the coast—but the expression of the Early Girl tomato is slightly different there. I find it impossible to choose a favorite without also acknowledging where it's grown, how it's taken care of, and when it's harvested. That's why I'm so often disappointed when I try to plant Italian San Marzano tomatoes here in Northern California. It might be because Italian farmers know exactly where the San Marzano grows best; after all, they have had more than three hundred years of agricultural trial and error. Food traditions are an important part of the preservation of biodiversity and terroir. Maybe there is someone in California who's figured out the right conditions for growing tomatoes like the San Marzano variety, but I haven't found them yet.

Carlo Petrini calls farmers "the intellectuals of the land." It would take a very long time for someone like me to figure out the perfect variety to plant in my own little garden: What will be most fruitful and delicious? What will flourish in this particular microclimate? That sort of delicate calibration is what conscientious farmers and ranchers do year after year, generation upon generation. This is why it's so important to support these farmers and ranchers. They have an incredible library of experiential knowledge about their terroir, and we lose this knowledge every time a plant or an animal is displaced by its industrially farmed substitute. This knowledge can also extend far beyond just the crops they choose to grow. The traditional hedgerows of England, for example, which seem like simple barriers between fields, actually serve as havens of biodiversity, where birds and beneficial insects can live in close relationship to the neighboring crops or the animals grazing nearby. Not only do these hedgerows encourage biodiversity, but they act as effective windbreaks and boundaries. Instead of fences, why not plant hedgerows around schools and other institutions?

Dan Barber, the well-known New York chef, is trying to offset the loss of flavorful heritage plant varieties by creating a seed company, Row 7, that works with a geneticist to cultivate and develop a wide range of vegetables for taste and nutrition. This goes directly against what industrial agriculture has focused on for the past sixty years: propagating fruits and vegetables for ease of transport and a long shelf life, and not for their deliciousness. At Row 7, they are growing squashes that change color in the field when they're really ripe, so harvesters know exactly when to pick them. It is a sort of virtuous genetic modification—the sort of careful, responsible, Mendelian hybridization we have been doing with plant varieties forever. But while it used to take up to seventy years to cultivate and develop a new variety, it now takes less than a decade, thanks to the use of digital sensors and computer technology that can identify the precise moment the crops are primed for pollination. It was a lesson for me how computer technology can be used in such a humane and organic approach to growing food.

⌒

Every September in Berkeley, I can't help sampling a few figs from around my neighborhood, because they're in season here for only a few weeks. Most of these figs never fully ripen, but on my walks I've discovered a nearby tree—an unknown variety with tiny, dark figs—that is divine. I've thought it was impossible to grow truly delicious figs in Berkeley because of our microclimate. But there's so much biodiversity that we don't notice, even in our own urban neighborhoods. Biodiversity is not just about undiscovered varieties that exist out in pristine, untouched wilderness. It can flourish right under our noses, in cities and suburbs and by the sides of roads. Biodiversity can exist in a field full of weeds on a vacant lot.

Tapping into that hidden urban or suburban biodiversity is a gratifying experience—and one that can connect us directly to our environment. Foraging has been part of Chez Panisse from the very beginning, and it changed the nature of the restaurant. Since the early 1970s, we have been collecting wild fennel down by the bay, using it to wrap whole fish, harvesting the seeds for spice mixtures, or drying the stalks and throwing them into the fire to perfume the fish. We forage other foods too: blackberries, nettles, purslane. You don't even know what's there until you begin to look. In the early days, we would forage mussels on the rocks up the coast. We've always foraged mushrooms, too—in fact, it's the only way you can find certain choice types. While you do have to be very careful about identifying them properly with the help of a mycologist, delicious edible wild mushrooms grow all around the world.

⌒

Mesclun is a beautiful expression of biodiversity. The word *mesclun* literally means "mix": the salad comes from a distinctive mixture of at least seven young greens that grow wild in the South of France: rocket (arugula), dandelion, chervil, frisée, and various types of young lettuce. The leaves are very strong, some of them a little bitter. I first tasted mesclun in Nice in the 1970s, which at the time was the only place this type of salad was served. In the United States, all we were eating was wedges of iceberg lettuce with Wishbone dressing—and perhaps a little romaine in a Caesar salad. When I tasted mesclun, I was astonished by the complexity of flavors and delighted by the delicious way they melded together in an anchovy-garlic vinaigrette. I was so delighted, in fact, that I brought seeds back from France, turned my entire backyard into lettuce beds, and grew mesclun to serve at Chez Panisse in its early days.

What's fascinating about mesclun today is seeing how salad has changed over the past fifty years as it's become more popular and demand has increased. It has been gratifying to see the way that the American public has discovered these varieties and learned to appreciate their flavors and textures. But even as backyard gardeners have begun planting these heirloom lettuces, big lettuce farmers have also seen that popularity, analyzed it superficially, and then packaged that analysis. This commercial mesclun doesn't have much to do with my little mesclun salad of the 1970s. The plastic-boxed mesclun mix you see in the supermarkets is not wild, or bitter; and it's not the unique and unexpected combination of varieties that all come together to create an utterly distinctive taste. I do have an emotional investment in this misappropriation. There are not many things I feel like I can take credit for, but I do believe the word *mesclun* came into the American vocabulary in part because of that mixture of lettuces we served at Chez Panisse—and still do. And I suspect that in some way I'm partially responsible for the fate of mesclun.

Preserving all these unique varieties isn't just a sort of dilettantism. It isn't merely about appreciating the beauty of different varieties or tasting new flavors. Crop diversity is central to food security. Climate change is already putting dramatic new pressures on plants, and adapting agriculture to our changing climate is of paramount importance. The more types of plants we have, the bigger the genetic pool we have to draw upon, and the greater the possibility that we will be able to find drought-resistant plants that can survive in the face of ever more extreme temperatures. This struggle to achieve true food security is one of the greatest challenges of our time, and we desperately need an understanding of biodiversity in order to maintain it.

⌒

The entire growth-and-harvest cycle begins, of course, with a seed. Saving and sharing seeds connects us to one another and is one of our most ancient practices. Because seeds are tiny natural libraries of genetic material, our lives depend on the seeds that are carefully preserved in seed banks all over the world. Those seed banks house thousands of years of agricultural knowledge, and it's critical that we protect them. Seed saving may be one of agriculture's most important missions right now. My friend the journalist Mark Schapiro, the author of *Seeds of Resistance*, told me that there used to be a very important Middle Eastern seed bank in Iraq. During the 2003 invasion of that country, there were bombings near the seed bank in Abu Ghraib, and the building was in danger of being hit. Iraqi scientists knew the significance of those seeds and scrambled to take them out before the bank was destroyed. They ended up transporting their seeds to another seed bank in Aleppo, Syria, which houses hundreds of thousands of seeds. Then the war in Syria escalated, and in 2012 scientists saved what seeds they could and brought them to a seed bank in Lebanon, where they are now. Recently, there was a drought in Kansas, which, alarmingly, is happening more often, and the University of Kansas was desperately looking for Middle Eastern drought-resistant seeds. And where did the University of Kansas end up getting its seeds? From the Lebanese seed bank. Seeds have always been shared. (At least, until Monsanto started patenting them!) Seeds are quite literally the source of life.

That sort of peaceful exchange is what happens every few years at Slow Food International's Terra Madre conference, in Torino, Italy: five thousand people from 150 countries gather to share their seeds, their farming methods, and their unique varieties of fruits and vegetables. All these participants are committed to preserving tradition and taste in the face of the fast food industry. It's an expression of global human biodiversity, too: cooks, farmers, artisans, and activists coming together to engage with one another and share their growing and cooking practices. Every culture in the world has a history of growing and cooking food for health, taste, beauty, and affordability. When we have cultural diversity on the plate, all these beneficial elements are strengthened—which is why we must learn about ingredients from different food traditions. Now I'm searching for the foundational foods of cultures all over the world, trying to determine what can be gleaned for our diets here in this country—especially for school lunch. There are many ways that other cultures can teach us how to get the nutrition we need at an affordable price. We need to figure out all the possible ways to address these issues, using our collective traditional wisdom.

Vandana Shiva, the Indian scholar and environmental activist, has said, "Uniformity is not nature's way; diversity is nature's way." I know she was speaking about agriculture, but that same biodiversity extends to us, to the human species. An understanding of the value of biodiversity helps us see that everything—and everyone—has a part to play. Biodiversity shows us how we all need one another in order to create something that's greater than the sum of its parts.

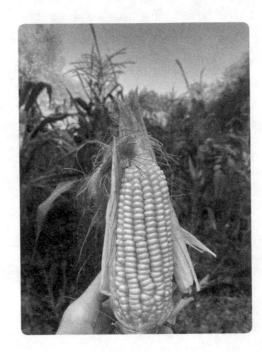

SEASONALITY

Seasonality means eating and living in rhythm
with the changing seasons. We are all aware of
the seasons and their impact on our daily lives.
But not many people understand what the
seasons mean for our food supply. When we
eat foods that are in season, we are connected
with the local cycles of germination, growth,
fruiting, death, decay, dormancy, and
regeneration. Understanding the seasons
teaches us patience and discernment and helps
us determine where we are in time and space
and how we can live in harmony with nature.

I n the very early days of Chez Panisse, I knew the importance of the flavor and freshness of our ingredients, but
seasonality wasn't uppermost in my mind. We'd have a chilled
soup in the summer and a warm one in the winter, but we
were more focused on following traditional recipes and figuring out what made a good menu. We had a different menu
every day, but not strictly because of what was in season. It
was more of an intellectual exercise: because we served only

one fixed-price menu in the early 1970s, we had to make sure it was interesting and different every evening so we could please the clientele. This was a big challenge. Back then, desserts were the arena where our cooking was more seasonally determined, though we weren't consciously talking about it that way at first. It was more along the lines of "Oh, God, the fruits that came in aren't good enough—we'd better make an almond tart instead." The truth was, seasonality was an invisible force out there that we were grappling with every day, but we weren't fully committed to understanding what it meant. At a certain point, instead of feeling limited by seasonality, we started to embrace it. We could focus on exactly what was ripe and perfect in that moment and surprise people with the taste of a fruit or a vegetable they didn't expect. It invigorated our daily menu, which is now entirely inspired by the seasons. I can't think of planning a menu any other way.

The shift to seasonal cooking at Chez Panisse came with our connection to the farmer Bob Cannard, and the aliveness of the food that came into the restaurant from his farm. In the late 1970s, my father and mother were tasked with the job of finding a local, sustainable farm to partner with the restaurant. We wanted a farm that we could rely on to provide a significant portion of the produce we needed every week. My parents visited at least twenty-five farms in the area and ended up choosing one: Bob Cannard's. When my dad first went out to Bob's farm, he looked out onto the fields and couldn't even see the lines of crops. What was Bob even growing? It looked like fields of weeds to my father, a man who had long prided himself on his immaculately mowed lawns and fastidiously weeded gardens. Then Bob took him on a walk through the fields, pushed the weeds aside, and unearthed a beautiful carrot that was unlike any other carrot my father had encountered. The taste of it was transcendent, and it changed my father's entire outlook on business and agriculture.

When we started our work with Bob, we were disappointed that we couldn't get things from his farm that we'd hoped to get all year round. We adapted quickly, because the ingredients we *could* get from him were so remarkable. Part of this was because of his semi-coastal Sonoma microclimate; part was because he knew precisely which vegetables and fruits he could grow successfully at different times of the year. He would send us vegetables we didn't even know were in season. Finding something in the winter like Bob's carrots or chicories—which were so beautiful and flavorful—was an edible education. His ingredients made us realize that there were new and different flavors to be found, whatever season we were in.

―

Ripeness is the key to seasonality. There's a subtlety to ripeness, and it takes discernment to know when something is ripe: the right amount of give to an avocado, the color of the shoulders of the Blenheim apricot, the scent of a passion fruit. You must look carefully, evaluate the flavors, and figure out the essence. I find that practice at the restaurant deeply stimulating, and I've gotten better and better at it over the years. It's an exciting and educational process to understand different gradations of flavors. Discernment is not the same thing as judgment; it's not merely *This is good; this is bad.* To understand ripeness, you have to learn through trial and error—you have to taste and taste again.

You really come to understand ripeness when you grow food yourself. People who farm or have fruit trees and vegetable gardens in their yards—or tomatoes or herbs on their fire escape—learn through experimentation, and after a few seasons they begin to figure it out. At the Edible Schoolyard, for example, the kids now know exactly when the raspberries and mulberries are ripe, because they've learned from exploration. Before they started school, they had no idea what a mulberry was! But when they come back to school in mid-August and go out for their first science class of the year in the garden, they go straight for the mulberries. Ripeness pulls them in every time.

People might think eating only what's in season is unfeasible, or means denying ourselves foods we have grown accustomed to eating all year. We have been conditioned to expect the endless bounty of summer foods through every season, even though that's simply not the way nature works. I say this all the time, but in truth, when all year long you eat those same second-rate fruits and vegetables that have been flown in from the other side of the world or grown in industrial greenhouses, you can't actually see them for what they are when they come into season, when they're ripe and delicious. By that time, you're already bored. You're eating in a thoughtless way. Letting go of this constant availability doesn't have to be restrictive. On the contrary. It's about letting go of mediocrity. It is liberating.

Another argument I hear against seasonality is that we can't possibly feed everyone on this planet if we have to survive on what's locally grown. I don't believe that. I'm convinced that using networks of small, local farms is the only way we actually *can* feed everyone sustainably. Yet I'm always told, "It's all very well for you to talk about seasonality in Berkeley, but I live in Maine. We have a long winter. What am I supposed to eat?" I recognize the challenge. And it is true: in California, some fruits and vegetables do grow outside all winter long. Bob Cannard's extraordinary farm is proof of that. We are lucky. But it is possible to eat seasonally in seemingly inhospitable climates. We are so unaccustomed to eating in season that we've forgotten the traditional ways people have preserved and cooked food. I am amazed by all the ways it is possible to capture seasonality: salting cod, curing ham, pickling cabbage or carrots or turnips, canning tomatoes or peaches—or cooking with all the heritage varieties of dried beans, lentils, pasta, rice, spices, nuts, and dried berries. As recently as sixty years ago, preserving was a skill that most families had. One of the few things I remember my mother did do in the kitchen while I was growing up was stock our New Jersey cellar for the winter with foods from our victory garden: winter squashes, canned rhubarb, applesauce. When you know how to cook and preserve foods, you can employ these ingredients in myriad ways. Freezing can also be used to capture a moment, as with stocks or fruit that can be made into smoothies and ice creams later in the year. Preserving food helps us all be less food insecure. And while I am completely devoted to seasonality and the primacy of localness, I do recognize the benefits of Carlo Petrini's idea of "virtuous globalization": buying coffee, tea, spices, chocolate, and other nonperishable goods from people in other countries who are using best farming and labor practices.

I am constantly inspired by other cultures and how they've eaten seasonally for centuries, whether in the mountains of Tibet or the deserts of Morocco. Living in the season is empowering—and there *can* be enough local food, even in the months when there are fewer fresh ingredients available. It's possible to prepare yourself. You need to have cool places to store sweet potatoes and apples and nuts. You need to have the forethought to capture and preserve the bounty of the harvest when it's at its peak.

Eating in season also challenges you to be inventive. I find I take much more care with ingredients when I'm eating seasonally. I'm more economical, too: I might candy the orange rinds instead of throwing them away, and I might make a broth using the green tops of vegetables and onion skins. I'm not as inclined to let things go to waste, because I know this is the one moment of the year to have that beautiful spring pea, or that September fig. I cherish it.

The good news is there are also many ways to naturally extend the growing season. This is not the same thing as shipping food halfway around the world or building industrial greenhouses that rely on the use of pesticides. It's a way of working creatively with our shifting seasons. We know from the farmer Eliot Coleman's greenhouse operation in Maine, for example, that it's possible to grow food organically all winter long. In Milwaukee, Will Allen is growing food on a massive scale right in the middle of the city, using greenhouses that are heated by the composted by-products from local breweries. In cold climates, we absolutely need greenhouses where we can grow carrots and salad and herbs in a warm environment. One of the most extraordinary organic greenhouses I've ever encountered is at the Ballymaloe Cookery School, in Ireland; the sheer diversity of plants in it is staggering. It is an organic laboratory. They have taken the local agriculture around them and extended it through the winter. There are still limitations, of course—you cannot have a ripe cherry from a greenhouse in January—but your options can be expanded through skillful organic, regenerative growing practices. And it can happen all over the world.

In 2008 we were asked to put on a dinner in Davos, Switzerland, for the World Economic Forum, which takes place in January. It felt important to me to get these global business leaders to pay attention to the possibilities of the local food and agriculture—I wanted to feed them an idea. I knew that there had to be something truly local and organic at that time of year; I just didn't know what it was. I was curious to know what people actually ate in the Alps in the wintertime. I enlisted the help of my friend David Lindsay, who had worked at Chez Panisse and was cooking in Zurich, and pretty quickly we found organic herbs and lettuces that had been grown in small family greenhouses. We sourced local cheeses from the surrounding countryside. We found kale from another greenhouse, which we used to make kale toasts in the fireplace. We discovered there were mountain goats, so we prepared a delicious braised goat. And the biggest excitement: We found a local apple that had been carefully stored since its harvest in the fall. This apple, the Glockenapfel, is an heirloom that has been grown in Switzerland since the 1500s. The London-based pastry chef Claire Ptak was with us, and Claire used those Glockenapfels to make the best apple galettes any of us had ever tasted. That variety had been utterly unknown to her, but the galettes she made with them were astonishing. These kinds of beautiful taste discoveries can't happen if you tie yourself to the predictable, familiar food flown in from far away.

I've also joined the chefs Joan Nathan and José Andrés in cooking for an event called Sips & Suppers, in January in Washington, D.C., that raises money to feed the homeless. Since we started the event more than a decade ago, the knee-jerk reaction has always been that you simply cannot find locally grown vegetables there, because they aren't available in the winter. But again, I've been consistently amazed by what's in the winter farmers' markets, mostly from organic green-houses, of course: beautiful cauliflowers, carrots of every color, squashes, chicories, and pears and apples that have been stored for the winter. The chefs who come from all around the country to participate in the event used to bring all their ingredients and supplies with them, and now they trust they can find winter vegetables, cured meats, and more when they arrive at the Dupont Circle Farmers Market.

The middle of winter is a time of reflection, a time when we often lose touch with what nature has to offer. In California it is also the time when Jim Churchill's tiny Kishu manda-rins from Ojai are at their most delicious. I've made it a point every year to gather as many of Jim's mandarins as I can and deliver them to friends. I call it "Kishu diplomacy." When people taste the sweetness and ripeness of that fruit at that moment, a flavor that's so remarkable in the dead of winter, they are awakened to the power of food. I give out those Ki-shus to remind people that I have an agenda.

Patience is obviously part of seasonality, too. I am not a patient person. But I still have to wait all year long for those Kishu mandarins—there is no rushing that flavor. Meats have seasons, too, though they can be harder to discern: the spring lamb, the suckling pig, the grass-fed beef in the late spring and summer. Honoring the cycle of the seasons is what motivated us, about twenty years ago, to stop serving salmon year-round at Chez Panisse. We had been using salmon from Alaska, serving it all the time because it's something everybody likes, it's easy to cook, and it felt local enough. We used it for all the obvious reasons. But year after year, we noticed how the arrival of our own local salmon marked a transition to more sustainable and better-tasting fish. Eventually we decided we'd buy only truly local salmon, when it was in season, from about April to September. Every year, we can't wait for the arrival of our California king salmon. But we do wait. And when it's finally in season, we have it on the menu all the time, and it is sublime. Most important, cooking like this helps us to remember that we can't expect the salmon season to be what it has always been. The local salmon's availability is different every year, because of global warming, overfishing, and natural environmental shifts. Two years ago, the local salmon was available for only six short weeks. We have to go with nature's ups and downs. And when we do, we become more attuned to the bigger picture of what's happening to our ecosystem, and we want to take care of it.

When I first moved to California, I didn't think that there were real seasons here. And I was sad that the weather wasn't more distinctive. Growing up in New Jersey, you just *knew* when it was winter: the weather turned cold, you got out your winter coat, the garden died back, you changed what you were eating. Seasonality connects you with the cycle of life and the magic of nature. Can you believe that the apple trees are covered in snow and ice all winter long, and that in spring their delicate buds still come out?

During the very last days of fall in Berkeley, I like to place a vase of beautiful yellow sunflowers on my table. And I like saying goodbye to them: *See you next summer.* I accept the cycle, and trust that they will come back again the next year, at some point. And there are other plants to welcome as the sunflowers fade: In November, we have big bouquets of local red pistachio branches and persimmon leaves in the restaurant. Something always comes; it's the rhythm of nature. It is stunning to be in a room where the warming aromas are coming from the kitchen—you smell the soup on the fire, the wild mushrooms on the grill—and then the foliage and flowers complement and reflect that warmth. You really feel that this is fall at Chez Panisse. Those red-gold persimmon leaves bring nature inside, helping you understand the environment and the culture in which you live. This reflected warmth grounds you, comforts you, connects you with change. Because it is terribly important that we accept change. Everything is different all the time—when we want the world around us to always be the same, we are swimming upstream. Seasonality helps guide us and propels us to embrace change rather than dread it. When you accept the seasons, you feel the ephemeral nature of each moment and understand how fleeting and precious life is.

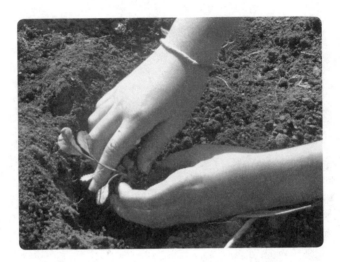

STEWARDSHIP

Stewardship is about taking care: taking
care of the land, which means taking care
of our whole environment—including all
plant and animal species and, by extension,
ourselves and one another. When we eat
with intention, we become stewards, which
changes our relationship to the natural
world. It's by becoming stewards that
we become true environmentalists. We
look to nature for guidance.

---

*S*tewardship. To be honest, I never really understood that
word. It's an abstract word, even when you know the
definition. It doesn't immediately conjure up a visceral feeling, in the way that *speed* or *cheapness* does. I think it's because
stewardship is not an outside force, coming at you, that you
need to deal with. Stewardship is more internal; it's about
attitude and intention. At its most basic level, stewardship is
simply about taking care of something, like a pet. You feed it;
you bring it in at night; you attend to it when it's sick. That's
what conscientious farmers and ranchers do: they listen to

the needs of their animals. They tend to the cows or the chickens they raise, in the same way that they take care of the apple trees or the lettuce they grow. Wendell Berry says stewardship "connects you to place." When you are a steward, "you are not a visitor, you get to know a place, take care of it. Without stewardship you are placeless."

I think, for example, about Wes Jackson and his project at the Land Institute, in Salina, Kansas. Wes is a steward of the prairie and has been studying how the prairie has an extraordinary natural resistance to environmental conditions like drought and fire. And yet when our current industrially grown annual crops are planted on the prairie and subjected to those same environmental conditions, they are destroyed. We tend to impose on the land our ideas of what we want to grow, but when we struggle to make those crops flourish, we look to pesticides, herbicides, and overcultivation. The mission of Wes Jackson's Land Institute is to learn from the way in which the wild prairie naturally sustains itself and has done so for thousands of years. He has been researching the prairie's perennial polyculture to determine why the hardy plants that exist in that sort of landscape are so successful. The Land Institute has been identifying edible crops that can grow harmoniously in the prairie environment, mimicking naturally existing ecosystems, without needing to be sprayed or tilled to death in the process. Roots that can reach farther down and capture more water and nutrients from the soil are among the drought-resistant adaptations of these crops. One time, Wes came to Chez Panisse and brought a plant with him that he had dug up from the prairie. He proceeded to demonstrate the depths of the roots to us by unfurling them across the dining room—and they stretched from one end of the restaurant to the other.

Creatively, stewardship is an entirely different stance than the one that's taken in fast food culture. Fast food culture ignores nature, forces it to bend to its will. In the United States, we work so hard to make things controllable, uniform. The case of the American lawn is a good example. How did we go so swiftly from victory gardens to manicured lawns that require the constant application of water and fertilizers and pesticides? Having a lawn isn't really taking care of nature. In fact, it's the opposite. As with fast food culture, you aren't working with nature; you're imposing something foreign and predictable onto it.

By contrast, stewardship is about being in service to nature, forging a relationship based on respect. Stewardship is about noticing the way a plant is evolving or changing. There is an openness in the attitude of stewardship that allows you to discover and reflect on the larger environmental patterns at play: Where does that water want to flow? What plants do best in this part of the field? The same thing happens in a kitchen: when I'm cooking, I never know what I'm going to cook until I see the fruits and vegetables from the farmers' market laid out on my kitchen table. I'm trying to let the ingredients speak for themselves, following what's ripe and in season and delicious. Here, you are working *with* nature—you're in a different kind of relationship, using nature as the primary model for how you do everything.

⌒

There's a radical cultural center in Arles, France, called the Luma Foundation, founded by the visionary environmentalist Maja Hoffmann. Within the Luma Foundation is a research project and think tank, Atelier Luma, which is a sort of product development equivalent of what Wes Jackson is doing for agriculture on the prairie. Atelier Luma investigates how to creatively use the local natural resources, gathering together scientists, researchers, artists, biologists, engineers, and designers who figure out how to manufacture objects that can protect the ecology of the Camargue region. They develop textiles out of local fibers, waxes, and resins; they're making the most beautiful, durable, Murano-style glass out of seaweed; they're crafting tiles and bricks out of local stones and shells; they're braiding local rice straw to protect against erosion; they're transforming vegetative waste into materials that can be turned into wall paneling and even lighting devices. There's a similar project in Finland called Spinnova, headed by two former physicists who, after studying how spiders make silk, applied those methods to wood pulp. Janne Poranen and Juha Salmela are creating a variety of usable textile fibers in novel and environmentally compatible ways. We can all be resourceful when we're stewards, and we can all help rebuild local economies. We can think like this in every small community in the country: How can we grow what's local? How can we find creative ways to plant our own gardens? And, beyond that, how can we produce all the materials we need ourselves, thoughtfully and respectfully, using the natural resources around us for guidance? I was so encouraged to read in *The Washington Post* that for only the second time in the past century, the number of farmers in the United States under age thirty-five is increasing. These farmers "tend to work small farms, grow organically, with a diverse array of crops and animals and are deeply responsive to their local food networks." This shift is happening all over the world; there's a new generation of farmers in Ghana who call themselves "agripreneurs" and who understand that farming is a forward-thinking, important profession. The value of stewardship is alive and resonating with the next generation.

Similar shifts toward stewardship are reinvigorating our city centers. Because the issues of urban food deserts are so dire, food justice organizations are coming up with ingenious solutions to fight back. In South Central Los Angeles, Ron Finley has been teaching people how to plant organic edible gardens in the neglected strips of dirt between curb and sidewalk; in the heart of Oakland, City Slicker Farms and the People's Grocery were both developed with the express purpose of taking care of the land and providing affordable, healthy produce to people in the inner city. Edible greenbelts—pathways planted with fruits and vegetables, meandering across cities and towns—become spaces that bring people's attention to food and spark conversations. The whole farmers' market movement that's now alive and well all across America is one of the fastest and most effective city-revitalizing interventions I know.

We can never underestimate the symbolic importance of gardens created by our civic, national, and international leaders. Michelle Obama's garden at the White House still sends a huge message about stewardship, community involvement, and childhood nutrition.

⌒

When we started Chez Panisse, we weren't exactly stewards of the land yet. If anything, we were more stewards of a culture, though we didn't fully realize it back then. We were passionate about the type of rustic French cooking that had existed for hundreds of years, and we wanted to preserve those ways of eating: how to assemble a traditional menu, how to cook what was fresh and in the markets, how to communicate those ideas to the public. We pored over the texts of old cookbooks, but in those early days we would always run up against frustrations at a certain point. We'd read a recipe from *Larousse Gastronomique*, which would simply say something along the lines of "Salt and pepper a chicken, put it in the oven, take it out, *et voilà*." We would follow the instructions, simple as they

were, but the resulting dish wouldn't taste like anything—
because the chickens themselves didn't have flavor. Pretty
quickly, we realized that the meats from local organic ranchers
were more flavorful—perhaps as flavorful as the meat had
been when *Larousse Gastronomique* was first published in France,
in the 1930s, before industrial agriculture took hold. We realized, too, that the flavor related very directly to how the
animals were being taken care of and what they were being
fed. When we changed from conventional chickens to pasture-
raised organic ones, the taste was dramatically different. And
the vegetables from local organic farmers tasted better, too. We
realized that we had to become part of the economic support
system that allowed these farmers to continue doing their good
work. As it turned out, we couldn't be stewards of a culture
without also becoming stewards of the land.

The ultimate stewardship we can practice in the restaurant is feeding people delicious food that's good for them, and
that has been grown in a way that considers the environment.
I couldn't imagine running a restaurant where you're not
thinking about that as your primary motivation, especially in
the face of climate change. When you're feeding people in the
right way, I think they digest stewardship almost sublimi-
nally. I've seen it happen again and again. They feel cared for,
they feel connected, and because it tastes so good, they feel
inspired to cook that way in their own homes.

Stewardship isn't something simply practiced by farmers,
ranchers, and people within the nature conservation com-

munity. Teachers are stewards, too. They are stewards of knowledge and stewards of the children in their care. Motherhood and fatherhood are forms of stewardship as well. It's the role of all parents. The point is, we are all already stewards in our own lives, in both big and small ways—so we are all capable of becoming stewards of the land.

⌒

Sustainability is a big part of stewardship. The basic concept of sustainability is that if you take something out of the environment, you put something else back in to replace it, thus avoiding the depletion of natural resources and maintaining an ecological balance. A sense of equilibrium, even fairness, is embedded in sustainability.

But, sadly, *sustainability* is a term that has been misused by fast food culture. It's been co-opted. I was onstage once at a Slow Food Nations event with Ron Finley. As we were talking onstage, the word *sustainability* came up.

"Sustainability is bullshit," Ron said. "What we need are regenerative practices, not sustainability." He explained that sustainability has lost its meaning as advertising agencies, fast food companies, and big corporations have begun touting their "sustainability initiatives" and accomplishments. What's more, Ron argued, the very definition of sustainability is about maintaining the status quo, and the status quo has become so degraded that what we really need now is *regeneration*. And Ron is absolutely right. We have passed the point of sustainability. What we need is regenerative agriculture, a way to repair the damage we've already wrought on our planet and on ourselves. This is a radical application of stewardship.

What, exactly, do we mean by *regenerative agriculture*? It's certainly a step beyond what we generally call sustainable. And it's also a step beyond the strict USDA definition of *organic*, which means no pesticides, herbicides, or GMOs. Regenerative agriculture adopts all of the values of organic farming, but it also focuses on the bigger picture of increasing plant and animal biodiversity, rebuilding the health of the topsoil, composting, and creating a functioning, thriving ecosystem. When you change field conditions and restore the soil this way, you promote biosequestration, the process of drawing carbon out of the atmosphere and putting it back into the ground. In the United States, industrial agriculture produces a large percentage of the world's greenhouse gas pollution, due largely to emissions from livestock and over-grazing: industrial animal agriculture is responsible for 37 percent of methane emissions and 65 percent of nitrous oxide emissions—two of the most prevalent greenhouse gases in the atmosphere. If we are to seriously address climate change, the food system has to play the leading role. Biosequestration is an effective, natural way to do this.

An essential component of regenerative agriculture is the understanding that the soil, like us, has its own sort of digestive system. In order to successfully grow healthy crops, you need soil that has all the necessary minerals, microflora, beneficial bacteria, and carbon—which constitute the food, if you will, for the soil itself. That perfect balance in the soil is critically important. Soil is naturally in constant flux, changing as nutrients are contributed and then taken away, but regenerative agriculture mediates those drastic highs and lows.

This is how regenerative agriculture links very directly to our health. When the soil is host to a wealth of beneficial bacteria, they surround and permeate the food grown in it. When you eat that food, these helpful microorganisms populate the microbiome in your gut. Scientists have proven that eating food that's been grown in rich, living soil can rebuild our immune systems.

Every culture in the world has thought of food as medicine: "To reduce inflammation, eat turmeric." "Whole grains enhance digestion." "Garlic is as good as ten mothers." But this emerging research about the microbiome, the immune system, and regenerative agriculture has been a revelation to me. We've always had an intuitive sense of the way food improves our health, but science is validating and confirming this in a way that makes it comprehensible. The soil gets healthier, the planet gets healthier, and we get healthier.

⌒

Stewardship is about regeneration, but it's also about conservation. There are so many wild spaces that I'm grateful for. Every time I travel up the rugged coast of California, I give thanks to the conservationists in the 1960s who had the foresight to protect it from development. Our wildlands need to be preserved for the sake of our collective human identity and national well-being, because wilderness has an incalculable worth that's greater than the strict economic value of the land. Even so, many of us still seem to think of wilderness spaces as separate from us—that going to them is like a trip to Disneyland, instead of part of something that we can participate in right outside our back door. But the truth is, we can have daily, positive, small, regenerative connections with nature in our own gardens, or on our fire escapes, or down the block at our local parks or community gardens. We can be conservationists in our own backyards.

One of the consequences of stewardship is that you become comfortable with nature. The idea that nature is forbidding and other instead of magical and welcoming is something people have always grappled with. But the beauty of nature is that it cannot be predicted. When you learn about nature, you appreciate the wonder and wildness and mystery of it. It teaches us to be present. It teaches us about ourselves, and our own lack of control of our lives. Nature is about the cycle of birth and death—and what could be bigger than that? We just haven't accepted that we are a part of that cycle. But if we can accept it, nature helps us to understand what it is to be human.

One of my most treasured books is David Brower's *Let the Mountains Talk, Let the Rivers Run*. Brower was the father of the modern environmental movement and the first executive director of the Sierra Club, in the 1950s, and he was instrumental in saving the Grand Canyon from damming in the early 1960s. He talked brilliantly about how the natural world inspires us and about our desperate need for "CPR": conservation, preservation, and restoration. I had the good fortune of meeting him for the first time several years before his death, in 2000, at the age of eighty-eight. He was living in Berkeley and gave a talk at Martin Luther King Jr. Middle School, where we had just started the Edible Schoolyard Project. After he spoke about the vital importance of CPR, he asked the audience, "How many people in this room would give up one year of your life to CPR?"

Almost everyone raised their hands.

"Well, I'm not going to be around much longer," he said. "Who of you is going to have the belief in your convictions to actually stand up and do something? Which one of you is going to take charge? If you have something that you feel that committed to, you need to take action *now*."

I heard him. And I believe if you have anything in your life that you feel that strongly about, you have no choice but to act.

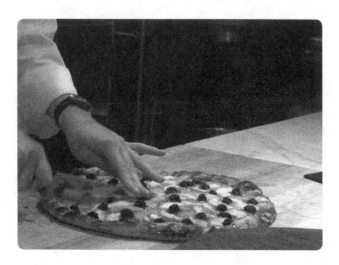

PLEASURE IN WORK

When we find pleasure in our work, we
see how jobs and tasks, even ones that are
challenging or difficult, can be done with
purpose and engagement. Work, a necessary
component of life, has the potential for both
ecological responsibility and a sense of dignity.
Finding pleasure in our work guides us in two
ways: it helps us recognize personal work that
is inspiring, gratifying, and productive; and
it helps us humanize any workplace we
find ourselves in.

When we hear the word *work*, we almost always have an instant negative reaction. We have been trained by fast food values like speed, convenience, and uniformity to expect work to be burdensome, something to endure, regardless of the costs to our minds, our bodies, and the environment—and something separate from the other aspects of our everyday lives. This can be one of the most difficult values to talk about, because it addresses how we feel about the jobs and careers we have chosen. Deep inside many of us is a feeling that we must sacrifice in order to make money and put bread on the table—and if we have to sacrifice our daily happiness in the workplace, so be it. It seems like that because we are living within a system that tells us work is drudgery. But that isn't the way it has to be.

The concept of work as pleasure is one I first absorbed during my early training as a Montessori teacher, and it was one of the most important things I learned from Maria Montessori's philosophy. "At some given moment it happens that the child becomes deeply interested in a piece of work," Montessori writes in her book *The Discovery of the Child*. "We see it in the expression on his face, his intense concentration, the devotion to the exercise." Work, she explains, might sometimes be difficult; at other times, less so. It is an ebb and flow over time. But on the whole, you should feel a sense of accomplishment from your work. There should be no underlying segregation of work and pleasure. In a Montessori classroom, any activities children choose to engage in are called "works," but there is nothing burdensome about them. Young children might be pouring themselves a cup of water, learning to cut fruit, setting the table with cloth napkins, making their beds, or sweeping the floor. They perform these practical life exercises with a sense of purpose and pride: they are gaining mastery over their bodies and their environment, following their instincts, and gravitating toward tasks that naturally interest them. And, most important, they are given the fundamental trust and respect of their teachers in order to gain that mastery.

A lot of these "works" are domestic jobs, tasks that are essential to living our lives. And we have been indoctrinated by industrial fast food culture to view these as menial and undesirable tasks, when in fact they can be therapeutic and empowering. Watering the plants in your garden. Cooking a meal. Folding laundry. Performing these small domestic tasks can be meaningful. Finding the pleasure in work is about sensorial experience and paying attention. Tasks like these help you see things you wouldn't see otherwise, and they connect us to our families, our communities, and the cycles of nature.

I have never thought of what I do as "work," in our culture's traditional sense of the word; I think of it more in the Montessori framework. Maybe it is a luxury to feel that way, but cooking is where my passion lies. When we opened the restaurant, I don't think any of us ever thought the cooking we did was that kind of work. Which isn't to say that it wasn't hard—it was. But we didn't think about it as going to a job every day. For one thing, we were still cooking the way we did at home. It was creative, and part of the joy was working together to figure it out on our own. We didn't have the usual industrial restaurant model in mind; none of us had worked in a restaurant before, so we simply didn't do things the conventional way. There was no hierarchy. We didn't have someone junior show up in the morning and prep the food for us—we saw tasks through from beginning to end. I've always felt that working with food is inherently pleasurable. And the restaurant was always mission-driven: we wanted to introduce taste and beauty to our customers in a very explicit, generous way. That idea of giving something to others was really what made our work enjoyable. That mission evolved over time to include the organic farming movement, and every time the mission expanded, we were galvanized and inspired.

At Chez Panisse, there is no real back of the house. In restaurant parlance, "back of the house" means the unseen people working behind a closed door: cooking, cleaning up the dirty dishes, dealing with the soiled linen, restocking the storage room. The back of the house is an area that's meant to be hidden from the customers. It implies that there are certain jobs that are distasteful to look at. I never wanted any part of the running of the restaurant to be concealed or unattractive. Everything that occurs in the process of running a restaurant needs to be examined: the waste, the staff meals, the locker rooms and offices. Every space and every job should be considered within the context of the whole restaurant. Yes, it is an aesthetic consideration, but ultimately it is a social and environmental one. If things and people are in plain view, you have to consider them. You have to recognize that those "unsightly" elements are part of the process—and question whether or not they can be made better, for the sake of everyone working or dining there.

One simple way to connect with the pleasure of work is to use your hands. Montessori says that the hands are the instruments of the mind, and handwork can be meditative, whether it's stitching, mixing ingredients by hand, or picking apples. That sort of work has a different character. There's a certain tactile connection when you do your work by hand—an engagement with the process, and with your senses. You become present and focused. There's a satisfaction that accompanies that engagement: the cracking of the egg is as much a part of the experience as the soufflé at the end. When you're process oriented—which you need to be when you're working by hand—you can also discern and adjust when things aren't feeling or working right. You can decide if you need to move more quickly, or slow down. You can adjust to your own pace. Take shelling beans, for example: you're figuring out the best way to open the pod to access each bean, and slowly refining that process as you go. And as you engage with the shelling of the bean, you're also noticing the way the beans pile up, and in the end you think, *Look what I did!* We have all our reservationists in the offices shell peas and fava beans and chickpeas as they take the restaurant's reservations. And what a wonderful thing to be doing as you answer the phone! Those staffers are participating in the creation of something that couldn't happen without their handiwork. We wouldn't even be able to serve fresh chickpeas or lima beans at the restaurant without their contribution. That task connects them to the season and the time of year, and the cooks are so grateful for their work. The cooks themselves also sit around the table at every chefs' meeting, topping and tailing beans as they talk through the menu for the day. Everybody does it together. One time, I put a basket of unshelled peas down on the bar upstairs in the café, and the customers started shelling the peas for us!

When you're shelling your own beans or peas, you also value them more: *It took this much time to end up with one little bowl.* You also understand the value of the person who might otherwise do that kind of work for you. Everyone should understand what it takes to pick beans in the field, or, for that matter, wash dishes in a restaurant. My father was a business psychologist, and he wanted to help our business work better. And in order to make that happen, he felt he needed to know what the dishwashers actually thought about their jobs, and what the work was really like. So he would go into Chez Panisse's dish room and scrub the pots with our dishwashers after hours. My father helped us change the way we operated the restaurant: we ended up opening up the dishwashing station to the rest of the kitchen, adding more windows, putting better ventilation in, and figuring out how the dishwashers could connect more with the cooks in the kitchen.

We rarely consider the actual physical environment of where we work. What's in the room? What are we looking at? When we were first setting up Chez Panisse, I was very

conscious of "preparing the environment," another important facet of Montessori's philosophy: I wanted to prepare the
room so that people would fall in love with their meal, and so
that we could all have a workspace that was inspirational. We
hung pictures on the walls in the kitchen, put up copper
lamps, placed special tiles on the walls around the sinks, and
hung beautiful old pots from hooks above the fireplace. I
wanted to find a way to bring the outside world into our
workspace, too, and it was always frustrating to me that the
cooks couldn't see the sun setting in the evening; there was a
wall between the kitchen and the dining room, which faced
west. Strangely enough, in its early days, the restaurant caught
fire, and that wall burned down. We never put it back up, and
now the cooks can see the setting sun every day. And the
customers can see the cooks at work.

In the winter of 2002, when we were initiating the Yale
Sustainable Food Program, we wanted to put together a special dinner at Yale to introduce the students and faculty to
the concept of farm-to-table. Michael Pollan lived nearby
at the time, and he offered to deliver the apples for the tarts
we were serving for dessert. (We're always using apples in the
winter, because they store so well.) But it was snowing hard
and he was late. In order to accommodate the late arrival of
the apples, we had to change around the entire way the university kitchen staff worked—so that when the apples finally
appeared at the last minute, we could stop everything we
were doing and all make tarts together. The kitchen staff had

never done that before, because the unions had strictly defined their roles and their pay: the person who does the prep
over here, the person who washes the dishes over there. As it
turned out, those collaborative apple tarts were fantastic—
the whole staff came into the dining room after the meal was
finished, and everyone cheered. Part of the pleasure of work
is breaking down those barriers. Our jobs are so prescribed
and we're so concerned with the money we're making that
we forget about the bigger picture of working together, the
joy and power of it.

⌒

Finding work that's pleasurable and meaningful to you is one
thing. What's equally important is making the job you already
have humane and enjoyable. But how do you transform a
work situation that's monotonous into one that's more fulfilling? My friends Davia Nelson and Nikki Silva, radio producers who create features for NPR, once broadcast a story about
the work of Cuban cigar rollers. These workers devised a way
to be entertained while engaged in the very repetitive task
they had to perform: A coworker who was good at public
speaking was paid to stand in the middle of the factory and
read to the rest of the workers. The cigar rollers would col-
lectively decide what they would like to listen to, and the
lectores would read them books that they otherwise might
never have read: Victor Hugo, Jules Verne, Alexandre Dumas.

The whole community was listening to literature together while they worked. That type of creative problem solving brings pleasure to work.

I don't mean that work always needs to seem blissful and easy, like being on vacation all the time. What I mean is that it should be engaging and fulfilling. It needs to be human. It needs to preserve our humanity, not strip it away. Our current models of the workplace came out of the Industrial Revolution. We are still following a nineteenth-century labor model. The conditions of many jobs have improved since then, of course, but that assembly line model has been replaced by a cubicle mentality: eating at our desks, confining ourselves to our own separate spaces, not thinking about how people can work together and interact—and, in fact, some jobs pit people against one another in order to maximize the company's profits. I recently spoke at Salesforce, the multinational tech company, and was asked if there was one humane step the company could take tomorrow to make a significant change in its business practices. I answered very quickly (and to no one's surprise): "Eat lunch together." It is important that there be a place for everyone to gather, sit down, share good food with one another, and have a conversation—not just with the people working at their desks but the people sweeping the floors or taking out the garbage. And the executives, too. There should be an actual mealtime, a proper lunchtime. Sitting down together dignifies everyone's job and expresses equality. I am always advocating for the same thing in the public school system: lunchtime should include the students, the teachers, the administrators, the maintenance staff. It should be a central moment in each student's day, a time to nourish themselves and connect with their whole community.

⌒

About thirty years ago, a woman named Cathrine Sneed called me. Cathrine worked as a therapist at the San Francisco sheriff's department, and she had witnessed firsthand the injustices that trapped young Black men within the broken carceral system. She had convinced the sheriff to allow her to create a garden at the county jail as a form of therapy that the men in jail could choose to participate in. This was Cathrine's way of fighting the system: she wanted to create a space for the men to be outside in nature that felt separate from the concrete prison yard. As a way to fund the program, she asked me if Chez Panisse would be willing to buy the garden's produce if it was grown to our specifications; I immediately said yes.

"Well, I'd like you to come and meet the students first," Cathrine said.

I tried to resist; I am ashamed to say I was a bit frightened by the idea of visiting the jail.

But she said, "You need to meet my students." So I went. Cathrine brought all the gardeners out into their seven-acre plot in San Bruno, right across from the main entrance to the jail: there were rows of six-foot-tall sunflowers, tomato plants, herbs, tangles of summer squash, a greenhouse. Cathrine asked the men if they would like to speak a little about what they had been doing.

One guy, nineteen years old, raised his hand. "Maybe I shouldn't be speaking up, because it's my first day in the garden," he said. "But it's the best day of my life."

Every time I tell that story, it makes me cry. Cathrine had had the revelation that helping to make things grow could be therapeutic for the men, and that working in the soil with their hands could be transformational. She understood that meaningful work in nature has the power to change your life. Not only did Chez Panisse start getting produce from them, but the program began giving the food it grew to the homeless centers in San Francisco. That was part of the transformational experience, too—offering food to others who were in need. Eventually Cathrine set up a transitional garden not far away, in the Bayview neighborhood, so that after her students left jail, they could stay grounded in what they had learned and have employment that they enjoyed. The produce grown there was sold at the Ferry Plaza Farmers Market, and the men who worked there often went on to work in San Francisco's Tree Corps, which takes care of the city's trees. Cathrine Sneed's Garden Project directly inspired me to start the Edible Schoolyard Project: if this experience in a garden can be transformational for men in jail, why not do it in the schools?

James Ralph Jewell, an educator from the turn of the last century, wrote, "School gardens teach, among other things, private care for public property, economy, honesty, application, concentration, justice, the dignity of labor, and love for the beauties of nature." It has been a long time since we last thought of agricultural work as being a valuable profession that needs to be taught in schools. Maybe we have never fully understood that in this country. There is a stigma around agricultural labor, exacerbated by our country's history of forcing enslaved people to work the land. It is a deep wound in our country that is being perpetuated in our current migrant farmworker and immigration policies. People doing that physically challenging work need to be lifted up—and paid accordingly. We need to understand that gardening and farming are fundamentally about nourishment, and that caring for the land is ultimately about our own good health and the health of the planet. We need to teach children in schools that farm labor should be recognized as dignified, honorable work that is good for our psyches and good for society. Agricultural work can be a higher calling. And the values that make this work a higher calling are the very same values that can be brought into any workplace, and into our society: connection to nature, community, nourishment, and collaboration.

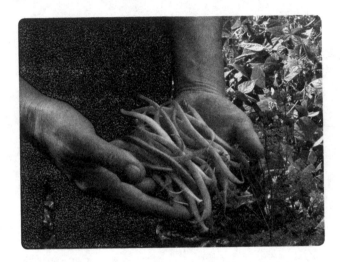

SIMPLICITY

Valuing simplicity is about cherishing the elemental. It fosters clarity, helping us cut through the confusion of our world, weed out the extraneous and the false, in order to see and connect with what's basic, authentic, and true. Simplicity isn't a denial of nature's complexity; it's an appreciation of its constituent parts. It's the opposite of more is better—a reminder that less is more. Simplicity encourages us to trust the power of the small-scale.

Once when I was in Spain, I went to visit the big central food market in Barcelona. I was drawn inside a little shop on a side street by the aroma: almonds were being roasted slowly over olive wood. I realized quickly that those almonds were the only thing for sale in the store. You could see the almond roaster turning the nuts in a metal barrel over the open fire in the back. They were serving them warm, in little paper cones filled to the top. I loved the single-minded focus of that shop: beautiful, perfect almonds, and nothing more.

I have always been drawn to simple cooking. But in the restaurant industry, there's a suspicion that "simple" means unsophisticated; it's what we used to encounter at Chez Panisse when French chefs would come into the restaurant in its early days and say, "A piece of fruit? That's all? That's not cooking—that's *shopping*." They were saying that our food wasn't complicated enough to be cuisine. But if what we mean by *shopping* is choosing the right ingredients, then, yes, it is about shopping! I never want to obscure the flavor of an extraordinary ingredient in an effort to make it feel "fancy." I like it when ingredients speak for themselves. And in order for that to happen, I have to see them on their own when they have just come in from the farm or market. Which leads me to provenance—knowing where the ingredients come from, one of the most vital things to me about the food we eat. Provenance, like seasonality, illuminates the taste of your ingredients. It guides you and educates your palate, helping clarify cooking and making it more straightforward. Knowing where ingredients come from helps you to know how to cook those ingredients (or how not to cook them). Should the fish be grilled? Or is it meant to be a tartare? There is always trial and error when you're looking to bring the ingredient forth, but if the ingredient in your hands is good and pure and alive, you can see and taste its essence directly. At home, many times the best thing to do with a great ingredient is the simplest thing: not much.

There are about a dozen basic ingredients in my kitchen that are the foundation of what I cook every day: Olive oil. Garlic. Vinegar. Salt. Lettuce and herbs. Anchovies. Spices. Flour. Eggs. Lemon. When I have those basic ingredients, I know that I can make just about anything.

In the early days of the restaurant, we were also criticized for having only one menu. But this was the only way I could simplify things and guide people toward what I wanted them to taste and feel and know. Now, people look forward to one menu so they can focus on tasting something they wouldn't have chosen for themselves, something that surprises and delights them, something they can savor and remember with clarity.

Simplicity has always been an organizing force at Chez Panisse, from how much silverware is on the table to how much food is on a plate to how each menu is constructed. We are always striving to make the entire experience clear, to bring the purest sort of understanding of food and its culture to the customer. It's not about avoiding complexity or inventiveness in cooking—a stock or a tart or a vegetable gratin can all be complex things to create. Whether the food you make is a traditional recipe or a completely new invention, it's about honoring the ingredients you're using, distilling their flavors in a way that feels true. When I think about a whole menu from beginning to end, I'm looking for balance. I think people are drawn to a plate where salad acts as a contrast to the crispness of fried potatoes and the tenderness of grilled fish. It's easier to achieve balance when you understand the essential nature of the ingredients.

⌒

I used to cook every year for a benefit in New York for Meals on Wheels, the nonprofit organization that brings food to people who are elderly or sick. We would go to Rockefeller Center, and chefs from all over the country would arrive and cook. It was all for a worthy and important cause, and the chefs were very generous with the food they brought. Restaurants were always concocting elaborate dishes, and the guests would walk around Rockefeller Center and take food from each station—it was a sort of high-end food court. But there was so much more than anyone could possibly eat, all in a jumble with everything else on the plate: caviar blinis next to cream puffs next to slices of filet mignon. So we decided that for our station, we would do something very simple: ice-cream cones. I also liked the fact that you couldn't put an ice-cream cone down; you have to hold it and eat it right away, or it melts. We made our ice cream from the delicate, prized Mara des Bois strawberries from the Chino Farm, in Rancho Santa Fe, and the list of ingredients in our ice cream was as simple as it gets: strawberries, cream, sugar, and that's it. But that Mara des Bois strawberry flavor was so intense it really took charge, and we didn't need to do too much to it.

We made our own ice-cream cones, too, which was rather labor intensive, but the result was deeply pleasurable. And the guests couldn't put their ice-cream cones down on the plate with the filet mignon.

Simplicity can also just be a perfect peach. What could be better? Twenty years ago, in *Fast Food Nation*, Eric Schlosser revealed that artificial strawberry flavor, the kind often used in fast-food milk shakes, contains almost fifty ingredients, many with names like amyl acetate, amyl butyrate, benzyl acetate, benzyl isobutyrate, and isobutyl butyrate. As a general rule, I feel that if you can't pronounce the words of the substances you're eating, it should give you pause. You shouldn't need an ingredient label for a head of lettuce or a bunch of herbs.

Fast food culture makes it impossible to understand what simplicity really means. It confuses us into thinking that simple is the same thing as easy and fast and convenient. Simple *can* be convenient and easy and fast, like cooking an egg or warming a tortilla—but I assure you that *simple* does not necessarily mean *easy*. In some ways, a loaf of bread is one of the simplest things there is: it's just flour, water, leavening, and salt. And a bread recipe can be quite straightforward. But would anyone call bread making easy? You need a lot of knowledge and practice and experience to know what bread making is about.

I use the phrase "less is more" all the time. I don't like to be served more than I can eat, and when I'm at Chez Panisse

I often ask for half-size portions because I don't want to waste food. At the Edible Schoolyard, we do serve dishes family style, but our objective is to teach students a lesson in portion size and consideration for others. That one bowl has to be enough to feed the whole table. When students serve themselves from that bowl, it is also a lesson in conservation: they are learning that resources are not unlimited, and it helps them appreciate what is on their plate. I'm sure they take that lesson home with them.

Simplicity in agriculture can be defined by small-scale farming, which allows a farmer to know the land intimately. The more you know about your land, the more you can bring out its fertility and productivity. You develop a closeness with it, and with nature. When you've walked the land thousands of times and seen it through every season, you know the potential and richness of it, even beyond what you have planted yourself: you know that the big oak over on the ridge is where you can find mushrooms in the fall, that the rocky knoll above the forest is where you can forage the wild thyme, that the watercress grows in the stream in late spring. Wendell Berry articulates this idea so well in his book *Think Little*. After walking his own land, he writes, "I came to see myself as growing out of the earth like the other native animals and plants. I saw my body and my daily motions as brief coherences and articulations of the energy of the place." It is incredible the amount of food that can grow on one small plot of land when you learn how to care for it in the right way. One of my mentors is the author John Jeavons, and I love the title of his book: *How to Grow More Vegetables (and Fruits, Nuts, Berries, Grains, and Other Crops) Than You Ever Thought Possible on Less Land with Less Water Than You Can Imagine.* The title says it all! When you think about it, a simple way to feed a family is to grow your own garden, even if it is not necessarily easy.

And sometimes, as the natural farmer Masanobu Fukuoka points out in his seminal 1975 book *The One-Straw Revolution,* the best way to care for land is simply by letting it be. Fukuoka referred to his method of farming as "do-nothing farming": He did not use machines or pesticides or chemical fertilizer or prepared compost; he weeded very little and did not plow the soil. "It seems unlikely that there could be a simpler way of raising grain," he writes. Yet despite the lack of these so-called necessary agricultural interventions, the harvests from his farm were similar to or greater than those of conventional Japanese farms. It's amazing that, nearly fifty years after the publication of Fukuoka's book, we are still fighting against this persistent mythology that industrial agriculture practices are the only ways to achieve high yields.

The "CheFarmer" Matthew Raiford and his sister, Althea, run a small family farm in Georgia (it's been in their family for more than 130 years!) that is utterly in the spirit of Fukuoka's agricultural simplicity. Raiford's relationship to his land is purposefully uncomplicated. This helps him minimize his farming interventions while clearing the space to witness his fields' natural balance and bounty. As he puts it, "Humans have taken so much from nature and tried to bend it to our will; if we don't like how it grows or where it grows, we just rip it out. But not everything is a weed. Take that simple dandelion: from the beautiful yellow flower to the dark chocolate root, all can be consumed and delicious. If we simply take our time, nature will show us how easy it is to live in harmony."

Valuing simplicity should be a priority when we organize our food networks. Local is simpler, and therefore more direct and responsive. Small farms are better able to satisfy the specific needs of their communities, and vice versa. It's a ground-up, self-sustaining approach to economics that avoids globalization and overreliance on corporations headquartered in another part of the world. Our country was founded, in part, on the ideal that the values springing from small farms and economies would best inform the values of a representative government.

We have witnessed this strength of smaller, scaled-down, decentralized networks firsthand during the coronavirus pandemic. The smaller farms have been the ones that are better able to pivot, adapt, and even flourish under new and unexpected circumstances. "This is one time where small is beautiful," our peach farmer, Mas Masumoto, said in a *New York Times* article in May 2020, two months into our country's quarantine. "When you're small you can make these shifts much more easily." We think we need these big corporations to feed ourselves, but we don't. And in fact, we have much more food security if we know the people who grow and produce our food—or if we produce it ourselves in our own gardens.

⌒

Living more simply can change your whole life; there's something powerful and liberating about paring down to the essentials. I think we actually crave a life without so much stuff in it and so many things to do. When there's less distraction, we feel less burdened; we flourish and have more energy. When there aren't as many things around us, we respond more fully to the world and to one another. Maria Montessori talks about the lack of simplicity in our lives by describing what it's like to walk into a big grocery store: we are adrift in the choices that confront us. It's a tangle of truth and falsehood, the authentic and the artificial. Simplicity is an ideal to strive for, because it creates a path for us that points to what is real and true. It leads us to honesty and integrity—perhaps the rarest values of all.

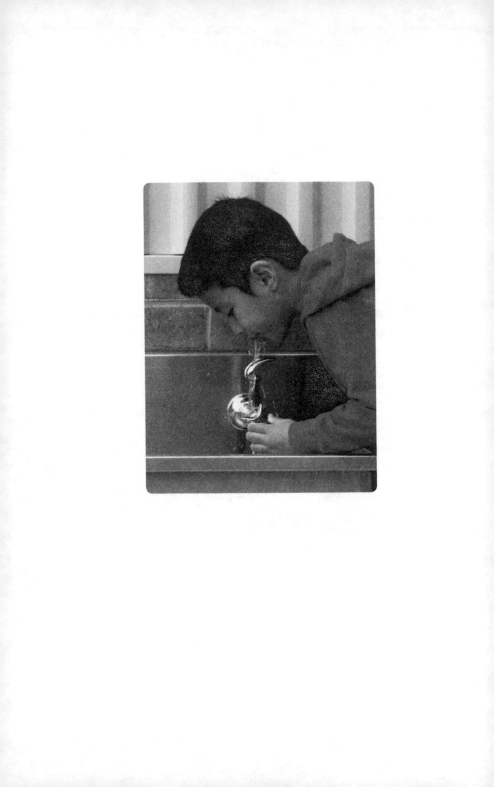

INTERCONNECTEDNESS

We think of ourselves as individuals, acting
on our own personal desires and impulses,
powered by our own unique wills. But
while there is an individual quality to our
experiences, we are also tied together—guided,
affected, and supported by a large, dynamic
network operating all around us. When it
comes to food, people who grow the food
are connected to people who pick the food
who are connected to people who transport
the food who are connected to people who
sell the food who are connected to people who
cook the food who are connected to people
who eat the food ... which is all of us. Once we
understand the ways we *are* interconnected,
to one another and to nature, a certain power
is unleashed in us that naturally leads us to
take responsibility for our lives, one another,
and the world.

I n the very early days of the restaurant, my friend Jerry was
delivering fish to Chez Panisse. One hot, sunny day, Jerry
was dropping off his fish and he smelled the garbage outside

in our dumpster. He opened up the big metal container and looked inside: the trash bags were getting holes poked in them by all the fish spines and fins, and fish were spilling out all over. Jerry was horrified. He marched into the restaurant and said, "Alice, you come out here with me." He took me out to the trash and said, *"Get inside the dumpster!"* And I did. I got into the dumpster full of fish guts, and I was shocked. I remember Jerry saying to me, "Would *you* like to be the garbageman who has to take this garbage out to the truck? Do *you* want to smell this if you're the garbageman? You have to think about the person after you." So I cleaned it out. That was for me the beginning of being conscious of how the entire operation of running a restaurant connected to the world—and also I became conscious of what, exactly, we were throwing away.

Ultimately, we changed the whole garbage system at the restaurant. We began double-bagging our fish, tying the bags up with string, and having two people carry each bag out and carefully put it in the dumpster. It was a real shift in our awareness. And after that, we became committed to composting and using compostable trash bags. Eventually we started sending our food scraps back to our farmer Bob Cannard. Bob wanted all the food scraps from the restaurant, including our fish, to be part of the regenerative agriculture process—food scraps that had originally come, in large part, from his own farm. Bob taught us that regenerative agriculture directly affects climate change: the act of composting pulls the carbon out of the air and back down into the ground, where it belongs.

Bob's entire farm is built on interconnectedness. When my father first met him and tasted that transcendent carrot buried among the weeds, Bob told him that the taste of that carrot came directly from the way he was farming. There was a connection among all the plants he grew next to one another: one weed might add nitrogen to the soil, one weed might fend off pests, one might hold the topsoil together in a certain way. It's called companion planting, and it works to nurture the health of the soil, and that, in turn, produces the most flavorful and nutritious vegetables.

⌒

When we first opened Chez Panisse, people brought food to us from their backyards: Meyer lemons, wild blackberries, radishes. I was so appreciative of that, because these gifts brought new tastes and ingredients into the restaurant, and connected us to our community and what was being grown around us. Once we started partnering with nearby farms, that interconnectedness helped me understand the true work that goes into growing food, and I felt an even deeper gratitude to the people who picked the beans and corn and strawberries, by hand, in the hot sun. I was aware of the restaurant's dependence on these workers—and I felt that they deserved all the respect and unquestioned support we could possibly give them. I felt so humbled. I still do.

This growing awareness of our connection to the land was happening in other restaurants around the Bay Area—and around the nation, too. In 1983, Sibella Kraus, who worked at Chez Panisse and was involved with the network of farmers around San Francisco, dreamed up the idea of having Bay Area restaurateurs meet with farmers for a midsummer dinner. The farmers brought all their ripe fruits and vegetables to us; we cooked their harvest, and then everyone gathered around a big table and talked about what was great, and what we wanted the farmers to plant more of the next year. Sibella named the dinner "A Tasting of Summer Produce," and I thought at the time that it was the most important food event in the country. We formed personal relationships with the farmers and with one another: the chefs learned how the farmers cooked a particular vegetable, what they loved about it, why they grew it. At that first dinner, there were about ten restaurateurs and ten farmers; three years later, there was another Tasting of Summer Produce at the Oakland Museum, and *three hundred* farmers attended. It was a groundbreaking event, one that united our restaurant community and solidified our farm-to-table connections.

This practice of tasting and honoring foods from organic suppliers has been carried on and expanded in the past ten years by Sarah Weiner and the Good Food Awards. The organization was founded in order to compare and showcase delicious products made from organic ingredients in this country. Artisan food producers from all across the United States submit their jams, breads, olive oils, beers, cheeses, and chocolates for review in blind tastings and are then honored at the Good Food Awards. It also becomes a forum where these food artisans from every state can come together and exchange ideas for the first time. We have never before recognized suppliers in this way; it's a whole new dimension of understanding taste.

Sibella started what ultimately became the Ferry Plaza Farmers Market, in San Francisco, a globally recognized model for organic markets. Models like this are important, so people can see the way it can work and bring those practices back to their own communities. I'm heartened by the growth of local organic markets all around the world. I often find myself thinking about what it's like for each farmer to go to a farmers' market: what it takes to load up the truck with produce so early in the morning, drive the truck two or three hours to get into the city, find the place to unload all your food, and never know whether you're going to sell it all or not. It makes me want to go to the market even in the rain. Because I am dependent on the farmers, and they are dependent on me. Farmers' markets are the best and most direct way for farmers and ranchers to receive the money themselves, avoiding the middlemen. And that's also the best way we, as eaters, can learn about farming, short of going out to the farm ourselves. When you're shopping for your food in that way, you start to understand seasonality and locality by experience, almost by osmosis. You understand interconnectedness just by going.

Community-supported agriculture has also been an incredibly successful way to connect farmers with communities. Through CSAs, you pay in advance for what the farmers will grow, which means those farmers are guaranteed a certain amount of income. Every week or every few weeks, you accept a box full of whatever the farmers are producing that's ripe and in season, whether it's Sungold cherry tomatoes and basil and plums in summer or squash and root vegetables and chicories in winter. A reliable local economy is created wherever these CSAs exist. The farmers are directly supported, and the community is nourished—it's a symbiotic relationship.

In the same way, schools are reinvigorating communities throughout the country, waking up to the idea that they can be beacons of education and also vital, stable economic support systems for local regenerative farmers and ranchers. This is what I call "school-supported agriculture." In the same way that community-supported agriculture pays the farmers in advance for all of the food they produce, schools can become similarly reliable and consistent buyers, paying organic farmers and ranchers in their area the real cost of food, directly, with no middleman. That's what Chez Panisse began to do almost fifty years ago in our restaurant community. School cafeterias are our largest restaurant chain, feeding thirty million

students each day. When all schools—including universities—
buy food *exclusively* from these suppliers, the real change happens. The regenerative growers win, local communities win,
and schools win. Students are immersed in slow food values
just by walking through the cafeteria doors.

⌒—

The ultimate form of connection, I believe, comes from sitting around the table with other people, eating together, and
sharing ideas. There is a research and arts institution in
Rome called the American Academy that serves as a home
for American writers, artists, and scholars. Since the 1893
World's Fair in Chicago, where the idea of the American
Academy in Rome was dreamed up a year later, the institution's mission has been to create a space for interdisciplinary
conversations and projects. But food was never considered
central: the food at the academy was like American school
cafeteria food—and in Italy, no less! So those who could afford to go elsewhere dispersed around town at mealtime. But
what better place to have a conversation than at the table for
lunch or dinner? That's why, about fifteen years ago, my col-
league Mona Talbott and I were recruited to reimagine the
food at the academy into something real and organic and
delicious—something that would entice people to come together every day, gather around the table, talk, collaborate,
and learn from one another's knowledge. Luckily, we had the

support of the president and CEO of the academy, Adele Chatfield-Taylor, who gave us the permission to go all the way: completely organic from the day we opened. We called this program the Rome Sustainable Food Project, and when we changed the food, it changed the whole culture of the institution. Scholars at the academy are now invited to work in the kitchen and in the garden, which gives them an entirely new way to think about the origins of their food. We also built a network of local organic farmers for the academy, centered around Giovanni Bernabei, the Roman counterpart to Bob Cannard, who operates a regenerative farm less than an hour outside the gates of the city. In this way, the institution as a whole became more connected to the landscape around it.

We were also interested in researching the old cooking traditions in and around Rome; those culinary roots and that history were so deeply felt in Italy, and were often passed down from mother to daughter. Tradition is part of interconnectedness—our connections with our histories, our ancestors, the cultures that existed before fast food culture. Oral traditions have been important ways of communicating and passing down food history from one generation to another. Even to this day, we never write down a recipe at Chez Panisse; it is always a conversation.

I know that there's a fine line between respecting tradition and feeling trapped by it: I lived through a revolutionary time, in the 1960s, when there was a rejection of many of our cultural traditions. I understood that impulse to throw out the values of the generation that came before. But we didn't completely reject tradition when we opened Chez Panisse, partly because we were all Francophiles. That tradition actually inspired us. Food and cooking are such visible parts of the history and culture of both France and Italy, and all of us had had an experience in those countries that had awakened us. It is also possible that we responded so strongly to those traditions because they weren't our own—and we felt free to interpret them without constraint. I felt so validated when my French friend Martine first came to Chez Panisse and remarked how she loved seeing French food interpreted with a Berkeley spirit.

With food, exploring traditions can be a tremendous learning experience: What flavor combinations have stood the test of time? We all felt that the past could be inspirational, not oppressive. It's nearly impossible to become a great cook without the wisdom of the past to help you. We saw the recipes of the old masters as stepping-stones to lift us up, and we never felt limited. And if we could come up with something even more delicious than those time-honored combinations, all the better. The secret is to be connected to your history and traditions without being bound by them.

Tradition also exists in agriculture—or at least it should. It's so important to know the history of the land, how the land has been worked, the possibilities of crops that people have grown before you. It's an enormous, vital resource.

Even the simple idea of a vegetable garden, the idea of

growing your own food, is about tradition—it's a mode of self-sufficient living that has been around for thousands of years. In countries all over the world, people grew their own food. When you grow food, you naturally want to keep that soil healthy. Cooking is really a tiny piece of the big cycle of the life of a plant—you have to choose the right seed, identify the right soil, take care of that seedling and that plant in just the right way, and know when to pick the fruit or vegetable. I think the whole growing-and-harvesting process is really 85 percent of what cooking is about. When you connect to the origins of your ingredients, it helps you to understand the entire cycle—how delicate it can be, and how linked we all are.

I've never understood how someone can call themself an environmentalist if they don't eat conscientiously. And vice versa: How can you eat conscientiously and not consider yourself an environmentalist? Wendell Berry says, "Eating is an agricultural act"—which of course means it's also an environmental act. And, therefore, eating becomes a *political* act, because every daily decision we make has consequences for the world at large. Every meal fundamentally connects us with life on the planet. Food connects us to the possibility and power of nature—the awe-inspiring gift of it. This is the place where we can make radical change.

CONCLUSION

How We Eat Is
How We Will Live

As I finish this book, COVID-19 is wreaking havoc all across the globe. Institutions and economies are in shreds, lives are being dramatically altered, many are sick or have died. It feels strange in this moment to talk about coming together around the table, since it is exactly what many of us have been forbidden to do. I can't help seeing this whole pandemic through the lens of food. The disease sprang from a food market. We ignored the ways in which animals are connected with one another and their habitats. Then the disease spread across the globe unchecked because of our denial of our own interconnectedness—what happens in China or Iran or Italy rapidly affects what happens in South Korea or New Zealand or Berkeley, California. Because we wanted all of our industrial supply chains to continue uninterrupted—because of those ingrained fast food values of speed, convenience, and availability—the disease spread further still. And the disease is being prolonged, to a great extent, by our misplaced trust in advertising—both as it relates to what we're told about the disease itself and the mixed messages about what to do about it. And yet still the fast food culture is relentlessly trying to profit, reinforcing and getting financing for the structures, institutions, and supply chains that got us here in the first place. The same ones that are pushing us toward climate disaster.

The silver lining, though, as in all times of upheaval, is that there is a real opportunity for alternatives. When systems and institutions break down and we come face-to-face with their flaws, we have the unique chance to reimagine them entirely. How can each of us bring slow food values into our daily lives? How can we bring them into the world at large as quickly as possible? (Because time *is* of the essence.) The most direct way—the most natural way—the most *pleasurable* way—is by changing the way we eat. Every time we sit down to a meal with friends and family, head to the grocery store, open a lunch box, turn on the oven, plant a seed, or get a snack at a concession stand, we have to ask ourselves a basic question: "Is this a slow food decision or a fast food one?" One of food's greatest potentials lies in the simple fact that we all eat. Each of us has the power—several times a day, if we are lucky—to choose which path we want to take. When enough of us change the way we eat in our everyday lives, the effects, as in any movement, will be monumental.

One of the most important things we have done at Chez Panisse is create our own alternative economic system. It helped us establish our own local, regenerative network that was more humane, vibrant, flexible, secure, and resilient than the industrial, scaled-up versions that existed around us. This sort of institutional restructuring has to happen everywhere for real change to occur. It is our most pressing, urgent need. And what better place to commence than in our public school system, with its immense buying power and educational potential? School-supported agriculture—with its centerpiece of a free regenerative school lunch for every child—is the alternative economic engine every community can embrace that would cultivate self-sustaining agricultural support networks everywhere and nourish all our students.

Gloria Steinem has written that public education is our last truly democratic institution. I know what she means. Every child goes to school—or should. School is the ideal place to reach the next generation the most directly, while they're still open and learning. Slow food values could be introduced naturally, democratically, and pleasurably in the course of every academic day.

The opposite of fast food scaling is the way in which edible education has already taken hold around the world. In the Edible Schoolyard Project's online network, there are more than seven thousand like-minded programs in schools and teaching institutions across the globe. The values of stewardship, biodiversity, seasonality, and beauty are present in all of the kitchen and garden classrooms. It is the transformational power of these values that students respond to. This is what we have seen at the Edible Schoolyard Project for the past twenty-five years. But these values are not owned or enforced by one person or one organization. They are universal, so schools create their own relationships to those values. They become individual organizations that are outgrowths of the community around them. In fact, regionality is essential to their success. The school and the program become better precisely *because* they're different from other schools and programs—because they are interwoven with their unique environments, climates, cultures, and traditions. This kind of network gathers the best practices from all these diverse cultures around the world, because it is imperative—especially now—to learn from one another's successes.

Let's be clear: This is not about regressing to some sort of idealized past. It is not a call to return to some preindustrial agrarian utopia that never really existed. It is about connecting to and supporting those who take care of our precious land in order to bring universal human values—through food—forward into our ever-evolving future. There has always been a farm-to-table connection. There has to be, by definition. We all get our food from somewhere, and always have. The only things that have ever changed over time are the answers to the questions of what farm, and what table. It is our dilemma every time we eat: What farm? What table?

What kind of future do we want to create? What kind of society? What kind of planet?

We can all rise to the occasion. Slow food values are our shared, natural legacy. They have power. And they are there just waiting to be awakened in every one of us. It only takes a taste.

Acknowledgments

This book has been a very long time in the making, and so many people have inspired it and contributed to it. Because it is very much a summing-up of my life's work, the people I should thank number not in the tens, but in the hundreds and thousands.

At the top of the list of people to thank are my collaborators and co-authors, Bob Carrau and Cristina Mueller. The actual composition of this book began more than ten years ago, when Bob started helping me write a stump speech that would make an irrefutable argument for slow food values and edible education; and in 2018, the three of us began meeting every week to wrestle with that argument and make it into a book. We had to dig deep into our own experience to find exactly the right language, and we agonized over it week after week. Without Bob and Cristina, the book would never have taken shape.

While we grappled with our message we got encouragement and assistance from my literary agent, David McCormick, and helpful suggestions from Jason Bade, Sue Murphy, Davia Nelson, and Steve Wasserman. When we finally had a manuscript, we got it scrutinized by my good friends Michael Pollan, Eric Schlosser, and Craig McNamara; and when they signed off, our opus got careful attention from the best of editors, Ann Godoff, who believed in the book right off, and from her associate editor, Casey Denis. Heartfelt thanks to all.

I owe an incontrovertible debt of gratitude to the many lively thinkers and activists who helped my ideas germinate, among them Carlo Petrini, Wes Jackson, Raj Patel, Wendell Berry, Michael Pollan and Eric Schlosser again, Helena Norberg-Hodge, Jonathan Safran Foer, and Mark Schapiro.

The deepest gratitude is also due to Bob Cannard, the Chino family, and Ron Finley for teaching me the real meaning of biodiversity and regenerative agriculture; to Jonathan Kozol, for exposing what he called the savage inequalities of public education; and to Esther Cook, for demonstrating the humane equalities of an edible public education, which she has helped bring to pass with the unwavering support of the board of directors of the Edible Schoolyard Project. That the project got under way in the first place is thanks to Neil Smith, the middle school principal who opened every door to us a quarter century ago. Since then, the concept of edible education has spread around the world, from the Edible Schoolyard Japan program at Aiwa Elementary in Tokyo to the école comestible movement in France founded by Camille Labro.

I must also acknowledge the incalculable contribution of la famille Panisse, the restaurant's extended family, now numbering in the hundreds, which has ever striven to live up not only to a gastronomic ideal but also to an ideal of working together in harmony.

Here I would like to slip in an extra thank-you to two of my oldest friends, Patricia Curtan and Fritz Streiff, both of whom have had a role in every book I have produced, starting forty years ago. None of the books—nor Chez Panisse, for that matter—would have been possible without Patty's creativity and aesthetic authority. For his part, Fritz has always been there to provide invaluable finishing touches.

And finally, my everlasting thanks to my daughter, Fanny, for validating the idea that beauty is a language of care, and for reminding me that edible education works.